A Color Hand

T0132741

Rheumatology

Ted R Mikuls, MD, MSPH
Professor, Internal Medicine
Division of Rheumatology
University of Nebraska Medical Center and
Omaha VA Medical Center,
Omaha, NE, USA

Amy C Cannella, MD
Assistant Professor, Internal Medicine
Division of Rheumatology
University of Nebraska Medical Center
Omaha, NE, USA

Gerald F Moore, MD
Professor, Internal Medicine
Division of Rheumatology
University of Nebraska Medical Center
Omaha, NE, USA

Alan R Erickson, MD
Associate Professor, Internal Medicine
Division of Rheumatology
University of Nebraska Medical Center
Omaha, NE, USA

Geoffrey M Thiele, PhD
Professor, Internal Medicine
Division of Rheumatology
University of Nebraska Medical Center and
Omaha VA Medical Center
Omaha, NE, USA

James R O'Dell, MD
Bruce Professor, Internal Medicine
Division of Rheumatology
University of Nebraska Medical Center and
Omaha VA Medical Center,
Omaha, NE, USA

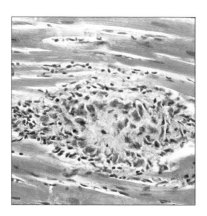

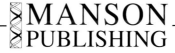
MANSON
PUBLISHING

Copyright © 2013 Manson Publishing Ltd

ISBN: 978-1-84076-173-3

A CIP catalogue record for this book is available from the British Library.

For full details of all Manson Publishing titles please write to:
Manson Publishing Ltd, 73 Corringham Road, London NW11 7DL, UK.
Tel: +44(0)20 8905 5150
Fax: +44(0)20 8201 9233
Website: www.mansonpublishing.com

Commissioning editor: Jill Northcott
Project manager: Kate Nardoni
Copy editor: Ruth Maxwell
Cover and book design: Ayala Kingsley
Layout: DiacriTech, Chennai, India
Colour reproduction: Tenon & Polert Colour Scanning Ltd, Hong Kong
Printed by: New Era Printing Co. Ltd, Hong Kong

CONTENTS

PREFACE

Arthritis and its allied conditions are among the most common causes of treatable disability worldwide. In developed countries, it is estimated that approximately one in three adults suffer from arthritis. The burden posed by rheumatic illness is formidable, not only in financial terms but perhaps more importantly in terms of the detrimental impact that these conditions exert on vitality and quality of life.

Rheumatology is the subspecialty of internal medicine and pediatrics perhaps most often charged with the diagnosis and treatment of conditions affecting the musculoskeletal system. Although musculoskeletal manifestations are common to many rheumatic conditions, these diseases are frequently characterized by multisystem involvement. To understand lupus or systemic vasculitis, or to understand the patient presenting with a complex connective tissue disease – is to understand medicine itself. The inherent complexity of rheumatic disease, coupled with rapidly evolving advances in care, mandates a comprehensive multidisciplinary approach to both diagnosis and management.

The aim of this textbook is to provide both a comprehensive and concise introduction to rheumatic illness. The contents of this textbook are structured in order to familiarize general practitioners, medicine trainees, and other ancillary healthcare personnel involved in the care of patients with rheumatic disease, with the major tenets of disease epidemiology, pathogenesis, diagnosis, and management in rheumatology.

CONTRIBUTORS

Jaclyn Anderson, DO, MS
Abbott
Abbott Park, IL, USA

Laura D Bilek, PhD, PT
University of Nebraska Medical Center
Omaha, NE, USA

Steven Craig, MD
Mercy Arthritis & Osteo Center
Urbandale, IA, USA

Annika Cutinha, MD
University of Nebraska Medical Center
Omaha, NE, USA

Brian Fay, MD
Avera McKennan Hospital & University
   Health Center
Sioux Falls, SD, USA

Michael Feely, MD
Westroads Medical Group PC
Omaha, NE, USA

Lynell Klassen, MD
Henry J Lehnhoff Professor
University of Nebraska Medical Center
and Omaha VA Medical Center
Omaha, NE, USA

Svetlana Meier, MD
University of Nebraska Medical Center
Omaha, NE, USA

Adam Reinhardt, MD
Department of Pediatrics University of Nebraska
   Medical Center and Children's Specialty
   Physicians
Omaha, NE, USA

Marcus H Snow, MD
Westroads Medical Group PC
Omaha, NE, USA

β2-GP-I   β2-glycoprotein I

AAU   acute anterior uveitis

ACE   angiotensin-converting enzyme

aCL   anticardiolipin (antibody)

ACR   American College of Rheumatology

ACTH   adrenocorticotrophic hormone

ADCC   antibody-dependent cellular cytotoxicity

Al   albumin

ALT   alanine aminotransferase

ANA   antinuclear antibody

ANCA   antineutrophil cytoplasmic antibody

AOSD   adult-onset Still's disease

aPL   antiphospholipid antibody

APS   antiphospholipid antibody syndrome

aPTT   activated partial thromboplastin time

ARB   angiotensin receptor blocker

ARF   acute rheumatic fever

AS   ankylosing spondylitis

ASA   acetylsalicylic acid (aspirin)

AVN   avascular necrosis

AZA   azathioprine

BD   Behçet's disease

BCP   basic calcium phosphate

BMD   bone mineral density

BMI   body mass index

BP   blood pressure

CAPS   catastrophic antiphospholipid antibody syndrome

CBC   complete blood count

CCLE   chronic cutaneous lupus erythematosus

CCP   cyclic citrullinated peptide

CD   (molecule) clusters of designation/clusters of differentiation

CDC   Centers for Disease Control and Prevention

CKD   chronic kidney disease

CMC   carpal–metacarpal (joint)

CNS   central nervous system

COMP   cartilage oligometric matrix protein

COX   cyclo-oxygenase

CPPD   calcium pyrophosphate dihydrate (pseudogout)

Cr   creatinine

CREST   calcinosis, Raynaud's phenomenon, esophageal dysmotility, sclerodactyly, telangectasia

CRP   C-reactive protein

CSS   Churg–Strauss syndrome

CT   computed tomography

CTD   connective tissue disease

CTLA   cytotoxic T-lymphocyte antigen

CTX   cyclophosphamide

DIF   direct immunofluorescence

DIL   drug-induced lupus

DIP   distal interphalangeal (joint)

DISH   diffuse idiopathic skeletal hyperostosis

DJD   degenerative joint disease

DM   dermatomyositis

DMARD   disease-modifying, antirheumatic drug

(ds-)DNA   (double stranded) deoxyribonucleic acid

dRVTT   dilute Russell viper venom time

DVT   deep vein thrombosis

DXA   dual-energy X-ray absorptiometry

EAE   experimental autoimmune encephalitis

ELISA   enzyme-linked immunosorbent assay

EM   erythema migrans

EMG   electromyography

ENA   extractable nuclear antigen

ERA   enthesitis-related arthritis

ES   electrical stimulation

ESR   erythrocyte sedimentation rate

ESRD   end-stage renal disease

Fab   fraction of antigen binding

Fc   fraction of crystallization

FCAS   familial cold autoinflammatory syndrome

FFP   fresh frozen plasma

FLC   free light chain

FMD   fibromuscular dysplasia

FMF   familial Mediterranean fever

FTA   free treponemal antibody test

FUO   fever of unknown origin

GC   glucocorticoid

GCA   giant cell arteritis

GFR   glomerular filtration rate

GI   gastrointestinal

GIOP   glucocorticoid-induced osteoporosis

GoC   gonococcal

GPL   IgG anticardiolipin antibody unit

HA   hydroxyapatite

HBsAg   hepatitis B surface antigen

HBV   hepatitis B virus

HCQ   hydroxychloroquine

HCV   hepatitis C virus

HD   Hodgkin's disease

HELLP   hemolysis, elevated liver enzymes, and low platelet count (syndrome)

HHV   human herpes virus

HIDS   hypergamma-globulinemia D with periodic fever syndrome

HIV   human imunodeficiency virus

HOA   hypertrophic osteoarthropathy

HPRT   hypoxanthine phosphororibosyltransferase

HSM   hepatosplenomegaly

HSP   Henoch–Schönlein purpura

HSV   herpes simplex virus

HTN   hypertension

IBD   inflammatory bowel disease

IBM   inclusion body myositis

IC   immune complex

IFE   immune fixation electrophoresis

Ig   immunoglobulin

IL   interleukin

ILAR International League of Associations for Rheumatology
ILD interstitial lung disease
INR international normalized ratio
IP interphalangeal (joint)
IVIG intravenous immunoglobulin
JIA juvenile idiopathic arthritis
KD Kawasaki's disease
LA lymphadenopathy
LAC lupus anticoagulant (antibody)
LDH lactate dehydrogenase
LFT liver function test
LGL large granular lymphocyte
LMWH low-molecular weight heparin
LPS lipopolysaccharide
MAC membrane attack complex
MAS macrophage activation syndrome
MC mixed cryoglobulinemia
MCP metacarpal–phalangeal (joint)
MCTD mixed connective tissue disease
MHC major histocompatability
MMF mycophenolate mofetil
MPA microscopic polyangiitis
MPGN membrano-proliferative glomerulonephritis
MPL IgM anticardiolipin antibody unit
MPO myeloperoxidase
MRI magnetic resonance imaging
MSS Milwaukee shoulder syndrome
MSU monosodium urate
MTP metatarsal–phalangeal (joint)
MTX methotrexate
NCV nerve conduction velocity
NHL non-Hodgkin's lymphoma
NK natural killer (cell)
NMES neuromuscular electrical stimulation
NOF National Osteoporosis Foundation

NOMID neonatal-onset multisystem inflammatory disease
NSAID nonsteroidal anti-inflammatory drug
OA osteoarthritis
ONJ osteonecrosis of the jaw
PACNS primary angiitis of the central nervous system
PAMP pathogen-associated molecular pattern
PAN polyarteritis nodosa
PCR polymerase chain reaction
PEG polyethylene glycol
PET positron emission tomography
PFT pulmonary function test
PG prostaglandin
PHTN pulmonary hypertension
PIP proximal interphalangeal (joint)
PM polymyositis
PMN polymorphonuclear cell
PMR polymyalgia rheumatica
PPD purified protein derivative
PPI proton pump inhibitor
PR3 proteinase 3
PRR pattern recognition receptor
PsA psoriatic arthritis
PSS progressive Sjögren's syndrome
(i)PT (intact) parathyroid hormone
PVNS pigmented villonodular synovitis
RA rheumatoid arthritis
RCVS reversible cerebral vasoconstriction syndrome
ReA reactive arthritis
RF rheumatoid factor
RNA ribonucleic acid
RNP ribonucleoprotein
ROM range of motion
RP Raynaud's phenomenon
RPC relapsing polychondritis
RSV respiratory syncitial virus
RS_3PE remitting, seronegative symmetrical synovitis with pitting edema
SAA serum amyloid A
SBE subacute endocarditis
SCLE subacute cutaneous lupus erythematosus
SD standard deviation

SI sacroiliac (joint)
sIg surface immunoglobulin
SLE systemic lupus erythematosus
Sm Smith (antibody)
SpA spondyloarthropathy
SPEP serum protein electrophoresis
SRP signal recognition particle
SS Sjögren's syndrome
SSc systemic sclerosis (scleroderma)
SSZ sulfasalazine
STIR short T1 inversion recovery
TAO thromboangiitis obliterans
TB tuberculosis
TCR T cell receptor
TENS transcutaneous electrical nerve stimulation
TGF transforming growth factor
Th1 T helper type 1 (cell)
TIA transient ischemia attack
TIN tubulointerstitial nephritis
TMJ temperomandibular (joint)
TNF tumor necrosis factor
TPMT thiopurine S-methyl transferase
TRAPS TNF receptor superfamily 1A-associated periodic syndrome
TSH thyroid stimulating hormone
TTR transthyretin
UA urinalysis
UCTD undifferentiated connective tissue disease
ULN upper limit normal
UPEP urine protein electrophoresis
US ultrasound
VEGF vascular endothelial growth factor
VQ ventilation–perfusion (scan)
WBC white blood cell
WG Wegner's granulomatosis
WHO World Health Organization

Overview of Rheumatology and Rheumatic Conditions

- **Introduction**
- **Synopsis of immunology in rheumatic disease**
- **Assessment of the patient with a suspected rheumatic condition**
- **Pregnancy in rheumatic diseases**
- **Pharmacological treatment of rheumatic disease**
- **Nonpharmacological treatment of rheumatic disease**

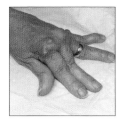
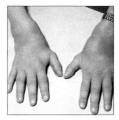
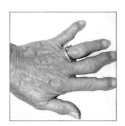
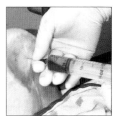

Introduction

RHEUMATOLOGY AND RHEUMATIC CONDITIONS – OVERVIEW

Rheumatology is an internal medicine and pediatric subspecialty focused on the diagnosis and management of diseases affecting primarily the joints and surrounding soft tissues. Rheumatic conditions are composed of arthritis and its allied connective tissue diseases. The term 'arthritis' is derived from the Greek 'arthro' (meaning joint) and '-itis' (meaning inflammation). There are currently more than 100 discrete forms of arthritis recognized, the most common being osteoarthritis (OA). Arthritis is often categorized by its distribution (monoarticular *vs.* polyarticular); its association with detectable autoantibody (seropositive *vs.* seronegative); or the degree of underlying inflammation involved (inflammatory *vs.* noninflammatory. (The latter is a misnomer since nearly all forms of arthritis are characterized by at least low-grade inflammation).

By the very nature of the multisystem diseases encountered in rheumatology, this is a field with multidisciplinary facets that include nearly all other subspecialties in medicine in addition to other major fields of study (genetics, psychiatry, surgery, dermatology, neurology, and so on). A review of the diagnostic criteria for systemic lupus erythematosus (SLE), a condition encountered in the rheumatology clinic on a near daily basis, illustrates the cross-disciplinary nature of this subspecialty. Major advances in immunology and an increased understanding of disease pathogenesis show that many rheumatic conditions can be characterized as 'autoimmune diseases' (autoimmunity can be simply defined as immune responses against 'self'). SLE, for example, is characterized by the presence of antinuclear antibody (ANA), while recent advances have shown that anticitrullinated protein antibody (anti-CCP antibody) are nearly exclusive to patients with rheumatoid arthritis (RA).

IMPACT OF RHEUMATIC CONDITIONS

Arthritis and its allied health conditions are highly prevalent with musculoskeletal complaints accounting for one in five to one in 10 of all primary care visits. Prevalence rates for different forms of arthritis and allied conditions are summarized in *Table 1*. The US Centers for Disease Control and Prevention (CDC) estimates that nearly 20% of American adults suffer from physician-diagnosed arthritis. Similar prevalence rates of arthritis have been reported from other developed countries. With an aging population, the burden posed by arthritis and its allied health conditions is expected to grow, with more than 67 million adults expected to have arthritis in the next 20 years. Arthritis and related conditions are the leading cause of disability in many countries worldwide (1). Arthritis and rheumatism, along with back problems, account for approximately one in every three cases of disability. Not surprisingly, the direct and indirect costs associated with the care of rheumatic disease are enormous. In 1997, it was estimated that arthritis and its allied conditions were associated with total societal costs of US $116 billion – 1.4% of the gross domestic product. With the availability of newer (and more expensive) therapies, these costs have likely grown. In addition to associations with

Table 1 Estimated prevalence of select forms of arthritis and allied conditions among adults in the US*

Condition	Estimated Prevalence
Ankylosing spondylitis	0.5%
Fibromyalgia	~2%
Giant cell arteritis	0.2%
Gout	~1–2%
Low back pain (lifetime, lasting ≥2 wks)	14%
Osteoarthritis (symptomatic)	12%
Polymyalgia rheumatica	0.7%
Primary Sjögren's syndrome	0.3%
Psoriatic arthritis	0.1%

* Sources: Lawrence RC, *et al. Arthritis & Rheumatism* 2008;**58**:26–35; Helmick CG, *et al. Arthritis & Rheumatism* 2008;**58**:12–25; Ward M. *Journal of Women's Health* 2004;13:713–8.

work-related disability and rising healthcare costs, many rheumatic diseases (e.g. RA, SLE, scleroderma [SSc]) are associated with increased morbidity and accelerated mortality.

MAJOR TREATMENT ADVANCES

Recent improvements in our understanding of immunology and disease pathogenesis have led to seminal advances in the management of the rheumatic diseases. In the last decade alone, there have been at least seven biologic, disease-modifying, antirheumatic drugs (DMARDs) approved for the treatment of RA, with many of these agents also approved for the treatment of juvenile idiopathic arthritis (JIA), seronegative spondyloarthropathy, and inflammatory bowel disease. Recent advances have yielded important alternatives for the treatment of end-organ involvement in SLE and, for the first time in more than 40 years, new treatment options are available for patients with chronic gout.

With the availability of a rapidly expanding treatment armamentarium in rheumatology, the importance of early diagnosis and intervention becomes even more evident. In this textbook, we provide an introduction to the rheumatic conditions, including concise reviews of arthritis and its many allied health conditions. The aim of this textbook is to familiarize general practitioners, medicine trainees, and other ancillary healthcare personnel involved in the care of patients with rheumatic disease with the major tenets of disease epidemiology, pathogenesis, diagnosis, and management in rheumatology.

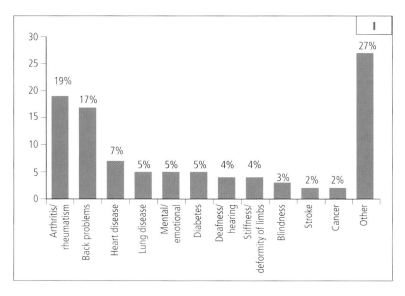

I Primary causes of disability among adults in the US, 2005 (Source: US Census Bureau, Survey of Income and Program Participation).

Synopsis of immunology in rheumatic disease

INTRODUCTION

The immune response is composed of antigen nonspecific and specific elements that can initiate the recruitment of cells and secretion of factors that induce inflammation. This process is efficient at removing pathogenic organisms (i.e. viruses, fungi, bacteria), but immune-mediated tissue injury can occur as part of this response. Moreover, dysregulation of the immune/ inflammatory response may then lead to the steps resulting in autoimmune diseases. Add to this the hormonal and environmental factors that influence immune responses, as well as the molecular basis of autoimmune disease, and the pathogenesis of rheumatic diseases is extraordinarily complex. This section provides an outline of the important features of the immune system, including some of its most critical cells and molecules, and the principles that relate to the pathogenesis of immune-mediated diseases.

INNATE IMMUNE SYSTEM
Definition

- No specificity to an antigen.
- No memory for an antigen.
- 80–90% of all immune responses occur through this branch of the immune system.

Mechanisms of action

Exterior defenses:
- Physical defenses:
  - Skin – epithelial cells.
  - Cilia – on mucosal cells beat outward.
  - Mucus – has a washing effect.
  - Stomach acid – pH 1.5–2.0.
  - Tears – washing effect.
- Biochemical defenses:
  - Enzymes – degrade proteins and nucleic acids (i.e. lysozyme in tears).
  - Sebaceous glands – release oils that are bacteriostatic or bactericidal.
  - Commensal organisms – 'normal flora' in the gut, vaginal area, other mucosal sites.

Cells:
- Phagocytes. While many cell types have phagocytic capabilities, the two major cells of the immune system that perform this function are:
  - Mononuclear phagocytes
    1 Macrophages – general term related to these cells throughout the body.

2 Monocytes – found in the blood.
3 Histiocytes – specific for a tissue.
  i Kupffer cells = liver.
  ii Microglial cells = brain.
  iii Synovial A cells = joints.
  iv Mesangial cells = kidney.
- Neutrophils
  1 Polymorphonuclear neutrophils.
  2 Predominant cells making up the white blood cell (WBC) count (~70% WBCs).
  3 Have granules inside the cell that contain enzymes.
- Recognition of 'foreign agents'.
  - Pathogen-associated molecular patterns (PAMPs) includes: sugars, proteins, lipids, nucleic acids or their combinations.
  - Pattern recognition receptors (PRRs) are the toll-like receptors or scavenger receptors.
  - PAMPs on a pathogen are recognized by PRRs on phagocytes that result in:
    1 Elevated microbial activity; peroxide, superoxide, degradative enzymes, and so on.
    2 Increased expression of adhesion molecules and co-stimulatory molecules.
    3 Phagocytosis.
      i The engulfment and destruction of the pathogen.
      ii Opsonization.
        a) Some molecules (acute phase proteins, i.e. C-reactive protein [CRP], serum amyloid A [SAA], mannose-binding lectin, and so on) attach to the surface of the pathogen (opsonins) and bind to receptors on the phagocytes.
        b) Results in an enhanced phagocytosis.

ADAPTIVE IMMUNE SYSTEM
Definition

The adaptive immune system is:
- Specific for an antigen.
  - T cell = T cell receptor (TCR, *Table 2*)
  - B cell = surface immunoglobulin (sIg) receptor (antibody that is never secreted, **2**)
- Capable of forming memory for an antigen.
  - First exposure primes the system with little or no response.
  - Second exposure results in increased memory and amplification of the immune system.

Table 2 Definitions of common immunologic terms

Term	Definition
Antigen	The whole material that induces a T cell or B cell response
Epitope	The part/piece of the antigen that the TCR or antibody recognizes
Antibody	A glycoprotein produced by a plasma cell that specifically recognizes an epitope on an antigen
T cell receptor (TCR)	Receptor on all T cells that specifically recognizes an epitope on an antigen (2)
CD molecule	Clusters of designation/clusters of differentiation: molecules on the surface of cells that designate the phenotype of a cell
	CD4+ = T-helper cells
	CD8+ = T cytotoxic cells

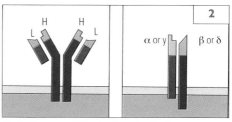

2 Antigen specificity in the adaptive immune system occurs first at the B cell and T cell levels. The specificity for B cells is conferred through the B cell receptor also known as the surface immunoglobulin (sIg) receptor. This immunoglobulin is surface bound and is never secreted. It is comprised of two identical heavy chains (H) and two identical light chains (L) that have an antigen binding site at the tip where these two proteins meet. When a B cell is activated through binding of antigen to this binding site on a sIg, the B cell under the right conditions will differentiate into a plasma cell and secrete antibody of the same specificity as the sIg.

The T cell receptor has an antigen binding site at the tip of one alpha (α) and one beta (β) chain. This type of T cell receptor is found on 90% of all T cells with the other 10% of T cells expressing one gamma (γ) and one delta (δ) chain. Regardless, activation of T cells results following binding of antigen to the binding site. Additionally, the T cell receptor is never secreted.

- A learned response that increases the specificity and memory of lymphocytes.
  - This is the concept of vaccination.

Mechanism of action
B cells
- Have surface immunoglobulin as a receptor for antigen made up of:

- Two identical heavy chains (one of the five classes, IgA, IgD, IgE, IgM, IgG).
- Two identical light chains (kappa or lambda, but not both).
- Inter- and intra-chain disulfide bonds giving structure and stability.
- When the B cell is selected, it will become a plasma cell and secrete antibody with the same specificity as the sIg.

HOW DOES AN ANTIBODY EXERT ITS BIOLOGIC FUNCTION?

There are two parts of an antibody (**3**): the fraction of antigen binding (Fab) and the fraction of crystallization (Fc).
- Fab portion binds antigen:
  - Antigen fits like a key in the lock.
  - There are sites where the epitopes on an antigen make contact with sites on the binding site of the antibody. These are called hypervariable regions.
  - Through this binding, the structure of the antibody heavy chain is altered and exposes sites for biologic activities to occur.
- Fc portion of antibody is responsible for the classes and subclasses of antibody (isotype):
  - Five classes of immunoglobulins (IgM, IgD, IgE, IgA, and IgG).
  - Subclasses for IgA (IgA1 and IgA2) and IgG (IgG1, IgG2, IgG3, and IgG4).
  - This portion of the antibody confers the biologic activity of the antibody.
    1 Opsonization occurs through the Fc receptor on neutrophils and macrophages.
    2 Complement can be activated by the Fc part of the antibody which results in:
       i Production of C3b which binds to the antigen and then to the C3b receptor on phagocytes.
       ii Production of all of the complement components and lysis of the antigen by the membrane attack complex (MAC).
       iii Crossing the placenta. IgG can, no other class or subclass can.

T cells

HOW DOES A T CELL RESPOND TO AN ANTIGEN?

The TCR comes into contact with an epitope that has been processed and presented through major histocompatability (MHC) class I or class II.
- MHC class II results in T-helper cell (CD4+) responses and results in the secretion of cytokines that enhance the immune response and direct other cells to perform their functions:
  - Activate CD8+ cytotoxic T cells.
  - Help B cells to class switch, become plasma cells and secrete antibody.
  - Activate macrophages.
  - Activate natural killer (NK) cells.

- Cytokine secretion determines the type of T-helper (Th) cells:
  1 Th1 = interferon (IFN)-γ, interleukin (IL)-12.
  2 Th2 = IL-4, IL-10.
  3 Th17 = IL-17, IL-23.
  4 T Reg = transforming growth factor (TGF)-β.
- MHC class I results in T cytotoxic cell (CD8+) responses.
  - Results in the secretion of perforin and granzymes to attack and kill the cell to which the TCR is bound.

T-HELPER CELL INTERACTIONS

CD4 on the T cell binds class II on the antigen-presenting cells. The TCR interacts with the peptide that is presented in MHC class II. Co-stimulatory molecules are engaged and the T cell responds (**4**).

T CYTOTOXIC CELL INTERACTIONS

CD8 on the T cell binds class I on the antigen-presenting cells. The TCR interacts with the peptide that is presented in MHC class I. Co-stimulatory molecules are engaged and the T cell responds (**5**).

Processing and presentation

Cells of the immune system present antigen to T cells by processing the antigen into peptides and placing these peptides into MHC molecules.

MHC class I
- Single polypeptide chain that has β2-microglobulin attached to stabilize the molecule.
- Binds peptides that are produced within the cell and puts them on the cell surface for CD8+ T cells to see:
  - Self proteins.
  - Intracellular parasites, e.g. viruses, bacteria
- Found on all nucleated cells of the body.
  - Includes MHC A, B, C, E, F, G.

MHC class II
- Two polypeptide chains (alpha and beta)
- Binds peptides that come from outside the cell (extracellular materials) and are processed (cleaved) in the endosome. The peptides are placed in MHC class II and then traffic to the cell surface to react with CD4+ T cells.

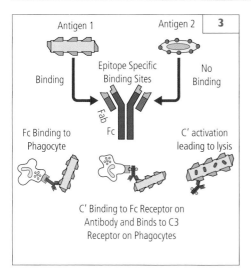

3 The body makes several million different antibodies that are capable of specifically binding to a wide variety of antigens. As an example, the antibody shown in this illustration has the capability of binding to antigen 1, but not antigen 2 through the fraction of antibody binding (Fab) portion of the molecule. Binding causes a conformational change in the Fc portion of the immunoglobulin, which is the part of the antibody that determines the class or subclass of the antibody. This conformational change results in binding to Fc receptors on host cells (predominantly neutrophils and macrophages) and the removal of the antigen. Alternatively, complement activation (C') can occur to initiate lysis through the membrane attack complex (MAC), or binding and opsonization through the C3b receptor.

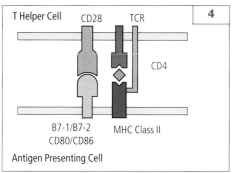

Antigen Presenting Cell

4 T helper cell (CD4+ T cell) activation occurs through an interaction with antigen-presenting cells that express MHC class II. Briefly, antigen-presenting cells take up antigen and process and present peptides in context of MHC class II. CD4 on the T-helper cell binds to MHC class II on the antigen-presenting cells, the T cell receptor interacts with the peptide in MHC class II on the antigen-presenting cell. Multiple co-stimulatory molecules are engaged (not shown) and the T cell responds.

- Found only on antigen-presenting cells, e.g. macrophages, B cells, dendritic cells.
- Includes anything starting with D = DR, DP, DQ.

Other characteristics of MHC molecules
- Polymorphic (i.e. multiple forms of the same molecule).

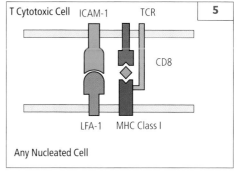

Any Nucleated Cell

5 T cytotoxic cell (CD8+ T cell) activation occurs through an interaction with nucleated cells that express MHC class I. Briefly, cells present peptides in the context of MHC class I. CD8 on the cytotoxic T cell binds to MHC class I and the T cell receptor interacts with the peptide in MHC class I. Multiple co-stimulatory molecules (not shown) are engaged and the T cell responds.

- Co-dominantly expressed (i.e. one gene from the mother and one from the father of each MHC molecule.
- Haplotype (i.e. groups of linked genes determined by mendelian genetics) used for:
  - Tissue transplantation.
  - Paternity testing.
  - Deoxyribonucleic acid (DNA) identification.

- Promiscuous. The epitope binding sites for both MHC class I and II are very 'promiscuous' and bind any and all (self or nonself) peptides that fit and interact with amino acids in the binding cleft.

Linked recognition

Linked recognition is a process by which T cells and B cells are able to recognize different epitopes of an antigen to generate immune responses. This explains how TCRs and B cell receptors can react to the same antigen without seeing the same epitope (**6**). Thus, the TCR and antibody see different epitopes on the same antigen which links their response to that antigen (i.e. linked recognition).

Tolerance

Since all immune cells produce their antigen receptors by spontaneous gene rearrangements, it is highly likely that they could respond to self proteins unless a mechanism exists to ablate this response (called tolerance). A loss of tolerance leads to autoimmune disease. There are two types of tolerance:

- Central tolerance or clonal deletion:
  - T cells:
    1 In the newborn through puberty, T cells that react to self proteins are deleted in the thymus.

2 After puberty, the thymus has involuted and this site is no longer efficient. It is thought that the liver and bone marrow then perform this function.
- B cells: occurs in the bone marrow.
- Peripheral tolerance:
  - Lack of co-stimulatory molecules.
  - Clonal anergy.
  - Cytotoxic T-lymphocyte antigen-4 (CTLA-4) or CD154 is up-regulated on activated T cells. It binds the co-stimulatory proteins B7-1(CD80)/B7-2(CD86) on antigen-presenting cells so that CD28 on the T cell cannot interact with B7-1/B7-2. Therefore, no co-stimulation occurs and the immune response is shut off.
  - Immune privileged sites exist:
    1 Sequestered antigens: antigens that cannot come into contact with T or B cells.
    2 Fas/fas-ligand. Activated T cells have Fas (CD95) that interacts with Fas-ligand (CD178) on the surface of target cells. This tells the T cell to undergo apoptosis.

Autoimmunity

The breaking or loss of tolerance results in the reaction of the immune system to self. Common components of autoimmune disease include:

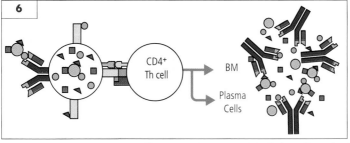

6 The surface immunoglobulin (sIg) on the B cell recognizes the circle epitope on the antigen. The B cell processes the whole antigen and presents the circle, triangle, and square epitopes in MHC Class II. CD4 (blue box) on the T helper cell binds to MHC Class II on the B cell (green box), and the T cell receptor (TCR) (purple box) on the T-helper cell recognizes the square epitope from the antigen that has been presented in MHC class II. With co-stimulation and cytokine secretion the B cell becomes a B memory cell (BM) and also proliferates to become a plasma cell. The plasma cell secretes antibody specific for the circle epitope even though the TCR on the T-helper cell recognized the square epitope. Thus, the TCR and antibody see different epitopes on the same antigen which links their response to that antigen, and this is termed 'linked recognition.'

- Sex of the patient: more often affects women than men.
- Age of patient: increased in the elderly.
- Environmental factors (e.g. smoking associated with rheumatoid arthritis and lupus).
- Genetic susceptibility: select MHC molecules (HLA-DRB1 in RA; HLA-B27 in seronegative spondyloarthropathy.

The mechanisms for evading self-tolerance to develop autoimmune disease (7) includes:
- Disruption of cell or tissue barriers (sequestered antigen release).
- Induction of co-stimulatory molecules on antigen-presenting cells following infection.
- Molecular mimicry (exogenous antigen that 'resembles' self-antigen).

	1	**2**	**3**	**4**	7
Mechanism	Stimulation of antigen presenting cells	Disruption of cell tissue barrier	Molecular mimicry	Superantigen	
Effect	Induction of co-stimulatory activity on antigen-presenting cells	Release of hidden antigens; activation of non-tolerized cells	Production of cross-reactive antibodies or T cells	Polyclonal activation of autoreactive T cells	
	Effect of adjuvants in the induction of EAE	Hashimoto's thyroiditis	Rheumatic fever Diabetes? Multiple Sclerosis?	Rhemuatoid arthritis	
Example			Antibody to bacteria cross-reacts with tissue antigens		

7 Tolerance can be broken and results in the development of autoimmune diseases through a number of different mechanisms. Normally, self proteins do not initiate the expression of co-stimulatory molecules on antigen-presenting cells which results in the inactivation of autoreactive T cells. When self proteins are present at the same time as some foreign antigens (i.e. infectious agents, chemicals), then co-stimulatory molecules may be triggered and T-helper cell responses induced (Panel 1). Some autoantigens are hidden (sequestered) from the circulation within tissues or inside the cell; if the integrity of these tissues or cells is altered (i.e. by infection, physical damage), exposure of the autoantigen and triggering of the immune response can result (Panel 2). An infectious agent that initiates either T or B cell responses might cross-react with self proteins (molecular mimicry) (Panel 3). Finally, infectious agents have been shown to contain superantigens that cross-link the T cell receptor to MHC class II nonspecifically (Panel 4), resulting in the polyclonal activation of T cells and the development and/or progression of autoimmune diseases. EAE: experimental autoimmune encephalitis.

- Superantigens.
- Regulation of immune responses –
  T-helper cell 1 down-regulates T-helper cell 2 effects and *vice versa*.
- Th17 cells: the 'autoimmune' phenotype.

Complement

Complement is the major mediator of inflammation (**8**) and initiates:
- Chemotaxis.
- Activation of mast cells.
- Phagocytosis/opsonization.
- Lysis of pathogens.
- Clearance of immune complexes.

Complement

- Consists of about 20 different plasma proteins.
- Makes up about 10% of the serum proteins.
- Is a major host defense system.
- Works in a cascade fashion.
- Is involved in the pathology of many diseases.

Activation (**9**) can be through the classical, lectin, or alternative pathways.
- Classical pathway:
  - Antibody:

1 One IgM antibody.
2 Two IgG antibodies.
3 Human imunodeficiency virus (HIV) and other retroviruses.
4 Mycoplasma.
- Lectin pathway:
  - HIV and other retroviruses.
  - Gram-positive and gram-negative organisms.
  - Arrays of terminal mannose groups.
- Alternative pathway:
  - Gram-positive and gram-negative organisms.
  - Fungi.

Function

- Lysis = MAC: C5b, C6, C7, C8, and C9 combine on cell membrane to form a pore causing the cells to leak and die.
- Anaphylatoxins = C3a and C5a.
- Chemotaxis = C3a and C5a.
- Opsonins = C3b.
- Complement system deficiencies can occur in different pathways and results in different pathologies:
- Classical pathway:

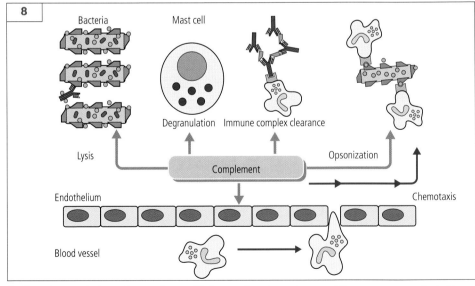

8 Complement is the major mediator of inflammation through many different processes including: chemotaxis of phagocytes, mast cell and phagocyte activation, increased opsonization, lysis of the offending agent, and the removal of immune complexes.

- Lupus-like disease.
- Severe, recurrent bacterial infections.
- Lectin pathway: recurrent neisserial infections.
- Alternative pathway:

- Severe, recurrent bacterial infections.
- Neisserial infections.
- Deficiency of C1 inhibitor: hereditary angioedema.

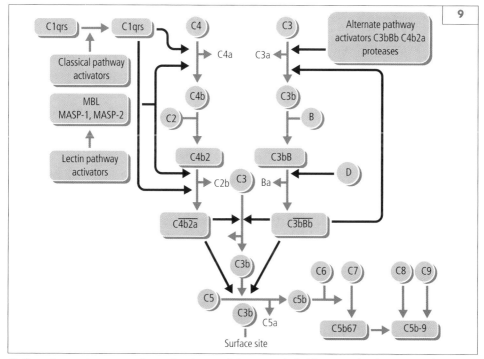

9 Complement is a group of proteins that work in a cascade fashion to make cleavage products having biologic and enzymatic functions. The major proteins are distinguished by numbers (i.e. 1, 2, 3, and so on) or letters (B, P, D, and so on); those that have been cleaved/converted (shown by the blue arrows) have suffixes (i.e. C3 becomes C3a and C3b).

Complement can be activated (activation pathways are shown with the red arrows) through three separate pathways; classical, alternative, and lectin pathways. The classical pathway is activated by antibodies (one IgM or at least two IgGs), the alternative pathway by the cleavage of C3 (bacteria and fungi), and the lectin pathway by various micro-organisms expressing terminal mannose groups (activation pathways are shown with the red arrows). Additionally, the C3b generated in the alternative pathway can bind more Factor B and generate a positive feedback loop to amplify the three activation loops. C3a and C5a are important in anaphylaxis and chemotaxis, whereas C3b is an important opsonin. If the process goes to completion, the membrane attack complex (MAC) forms resulting in the formation of pores, cell leakage, and death (lysis). Complement deficiencies may result in a number of different disease states including lupus-like disease and recurrent bacterial infections.

THE 'HYPERSENSITIVITIES'

The immune system has been shown to work by four basic mechanisms. Importantly, although they can be classified separately, they do not always work in an isolated fashion.

Type I (immediate) hypersensitivity

- Develops within minutes of exposure to antigen.
- Dependent upon activation of mast cells and the release of mediators of acute inflammation.
- Antigen cross-links IgE on the mast cell via surface Fcε receptor. The mast cell degranulates releasing:
  - Vasoactive amines.
  - Prostaglandins and leukotrienes are produced by arachidonic acid metabolism; results in a delayed component of this response that occurs several hours after the original antigen exposure.
- Can result in:
  - Allergic asthma.
  - Hay fever.
  - Eczema.
  - Urticaria.
  - Shock and even death.

Type II (antibody-mediated) hypersensitivity

- Develops following the binding of antibody to cell surface antigens. This binding can initiate:
  - Antibody-dependent cellular cytotoxicity (ADCC) by killer cells.
  - Complement-mediated lysis.
- Can result in:
  - Removal of the offending pathogen or foreign agent.
  - Autoimmune or inflammatory diseases:
    1 Transfusion reactions.
    2 Hemolytic disease of the newborn.
    3 Myasthenia gravis.
    4 Other antibody-mediated autoimmune diseases.

Type III (immune complex-mediated) hypersensitivity

- Develops following the deposition of antigen/antibody (immune) complexes in the tissue or blood vessels.
- Activation of complement attracts polymorphonuclear leukocytes to the area resulting in local damage.
- These conditions are all caused by high antigen load (persistent antigen) due to a weak or ineffective antibody response.
- Can result in:
  - Normal removal of pathogens or foreign agents.
  - Arthus reaction: pre-formed antibody reacts with antigen at the site of vaccination.
  - Autoimmune disease: extrinsic allergic alveolitis from inhaled persistent antigens.

Type IV (delayed) hypersensitivity

- Develops 24–72 hours after encountering the antigen.
- Only one of the four hypersensitivities that is T cell-mediated:
  - Release cytokines which attracts macrophages.
  - Macrophages activated at the site and produce tissue damage.
  - Under persistent activation this may cause granuloma formation.
- Can result in:
  - Removal of intracellular pathogens or foreign agents.
  - Contact hypersensitivity, e.g. poison ivy, poison oak, nickel, and so on.
  - Tuberculin reactions = response to purified protein derivative (PPD) test for tuberculosis (TB)
  - Granulomas (e.g. chronic infections, TB, blastomycosis, coccidioidimycosis).

Assessment of the patient with a suspected rheumatic condition

HISTORY

The diagnosis of rheumatic diseases requires a thorough history to identify clues to the appropriate diagnosis. It is helpful to differentiate acute from chronic, monarticular from poly-articular, joint distribution, and demographic indicators which may help to elucidate the diagnosis. Acute onset of symptoms usually suggests trauma, infectious-or crystal-induced disease. Chronic rheumatic disorders such as RA and OA usually present with an indolent course and are not typically associated with acute complaints. Systemic lupus may present with an acute onset of arthritis, but the multisystem nature of complaints usually helps to identify the correct diagnosis.

Monarticular disease is most commonly associated with periarticular processes such as bursitis, tendinitis, or trigger points. However, acute signs of inflammation should raise suspicion for crystal-induced disease such as gout or pseudo-gout as well as septic arthritis. In this case, aspiration of synovial fluid is necessary to make the correct diagnosis.

Polyarticular complaints of short duration are usually associated with a viral syndrome, bacterial illness, or drug reaction. When present for more than 6 weeks, suspicion for rheumatoid and other types of chronic arthritis should increase. An algorithm outlining an approach to patients with articular complaints is shown in **10**. Involvement of the distal interphalangeal (DIP) joints of the hands and the first carpal–metacarpal (CMC) joint is very characteristic of OA. Bilateral temporo-mandibular joint involvement in the absence of oropharyngeal pathology highly suggests RA. Lower extremity predominance of findings is suggestive of seronegative spondyloarthropathies and gout.

A complete review of systems is taken to identify symptoms of possible connective tissue diseases. The clinician should ask about skin rash, photosensitivity, sicca syndrome, oral ulcerations, symptoms of serositis, unexplained arrhythmias, renal involvement, neurologic complaints, and so on. Certain illnesses are more common in women (RA, connective tissue diseases [CTDs] such as systemic lupus, and fibromyalgia). Men have a higher incidence of seronegative spondylo-arthropathies such as reactive arthritis, and gout. Older individuals are more likely to have gout, degenerative joint disease (DJD), temporal arteritis, or OA while younger individuals may have trauma, infectious causes, RA, or fibro-myalgia.

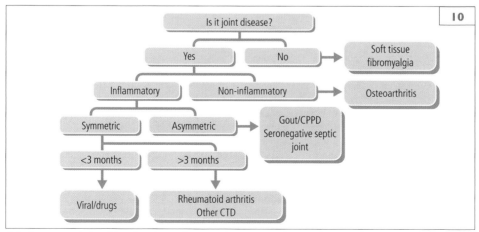

10 A proposed algorithm for the evaluation of patients with articular complaints.

MUSCULOSKELETAL EXAMINATION

A thorough examination of the musculoskeletal system as part of the complete physical examination will help to identify the correct diagnosis. Examination for trigger points, synovitis, joint effusions, range of motion, muscle strength, and neurologic findings should be done. Firm pressure on the joints and trigger point areas is necessary to identify tenderness. Comparison with the opposite side is important. Inflammatory diseases will demonstrate the classic signs of inflammation. Synovitis is described as a 'boggy' feeling at the joint line (**11**). Swelling of the joint may be due to synovitis or joint fluid. It may be difficult to separate these two entities. A fluid wave or ballottement may be demonstrated when excessive joint fluid is present. Bony enlargement of the joints is usually a sign of chronic disease such as OA (**12**).

Examination for classic deformities is also helpful. Osteoarthritic changes of the DIP joints (Heberden's nodes) contrast with the soft tissue swelling of the metacarpal–phalangeal (MCP) and proximal interphalangeal (PIP) joints that is characteristic of RA. Ulnar deviation of the MCP joints can be found in RA and systemic lupus. Swan neck deformities of the fingers (proximal extension and distal flexion) and Boutonnière deformities (proximal flexion with distal extension) are both characteristic of RA (**13**).

LABORATORY TESTING

Laboratory testing can be useful to confirm the clinical diagnosis. Some of the tests that are performed are relatively specific for a diagnosis but most tests are not. Some tests provide prognostic information and can be used to predict the disease course. Most tests are consistent with the diagnosis and provide little additional diagnostic information. Anemia, thrombocytopenia, evidence for renal insufficiency by elevated serum creatinine, and abnormal urinalysis with red cells or proteinuria indicate major organ involvement, but do not necessarily suggest a specific rheumatic disease diagnosis. An elevated serum uric acid may be found in gout but is not diagnostic in and of itself. An increased creatine phosphokinase level is suggestive of muscle damage from dermato/polymyositis, but may be seen with rhabdomyolysis; myocardial damage; drug-induced myopathy; thyroid disease; and in young, healthy African-American males.

Laboratory indicators of inflammation (acute phase reactants) are generally helpful in documenting and following disease activity. Useful tests are the erythrocyte sedimentation rate (ESR) and the CRP which is generally up to 100 times more sensitive than the ESR. If normal, these tests can be quite helpful in the fibromyalgia patient who has inflammatory symptoms without objective evidence of inflammation on physical examination. The differential of an elevated ESR is quite extensive and by itself is not very useful. When the ESR is quite high (>100 mm/hour), the differential diagnosis is more limited. The differential diagnosis for marked elevation in ESR (>100 mm/hour) includes:

- Malignancy (particularly multiple myeloma).
- Temporal arteritis.
- Chronic infections (such as TB, osteomyelitis, and fungal disease).
- Acute connective tissue diseases.

In general, the ESR or CRP is not helpful in following disease activity with the noticeable exceptions of polymyalgia rheumatica and Wegener's granulomatosis.

Serological markers are commonly used to confirm the clinical diagnosis. Rheumatoid factor (RF), an IgM antibody to IgG, is neither sensitive nor specific for RA. High titer positivity is more likely to be suggestive of RA. Recently, the cyclic citrullinated peptide (CCP) antibody has been found to be somewhat more sensitive (although similar to RF in some reports) and relatively specific for RA. Serum complement levels may be decreased with diseases that activate antigen–antibody reactions but are non diagnostic for specific disease processes.

ANA testing is widely used in the evaluation of various rheumatic diseases but is rarely diagnostic by itself. ANA positivity is found in many connective tissue diseases. More specific subsets of the antibody are often ordered as these subsets may be more specific than the ANA by itself. Antidouble-stranded DNA and Smith (Sm) antibodies are relatively specific for systemic lupus but are relatively insensitive. Anticytoplasmic antibodies are found most commonly in patients with vasculitis such as Wegener's granulomatosis. Details about antibody testing are provided in the chapters for each specific disease process.

ARTHROCENTESIS AND SYNOVIAL FLUID TESTING

Arthrocentesis with laboratory evaluation of joint fluid and intraarticular injection of medications is a valuable diagnostic and therapeutic intervention in rheumatology. As a general rule, patients who present with a monarticular complaint will likely need a diagnostic arthrocentesis to identify an infectious or crystal etiology for the problem (**14**). A thorough knowledge of the anatomy of the involved joint is necessary to determine the location for the arthrocentesis. Avoidance of major neurovascular structures is imperative.

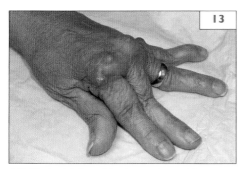

11 Synovitis of the wrists and small joints of the hands in a patient with inflammatory arthritis.

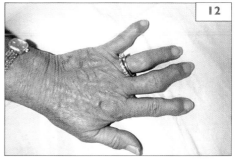

12 Bony enlargement of the PIPs and DIPs in a patient with diffuse osteoarthritis.

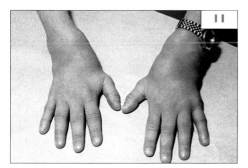

13 Marked deformities in a patient with advanced rheumatoid arthritis including ulnar drift, palmar subluxation of the MCPs, subcutaneous nodules and 'swan-necking' (most obvious in fifth digit).

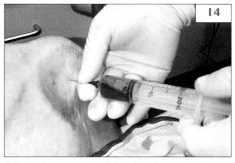

14 Arthrocentesis of the glenohumeral joint.

Ultrasound imaging may help with small joint aspiration and injection. Aspirated fluid should be routinely sent for total WBC count and differential, Gram stain, culture and sensitivity, and crystal examination (**15**). Other laboratory testing of fluid is not helpful. Removal of fluid can reduce pressure on the joint and relieve symptoms for the patient.

Normal joint fluid has less than 200 WBCs with a predominance of mononuclear forms. Degenerative arthritis generally has WBC counts of 200–2000. Counts between 2000 and 50 000 are characteristic of inflammatory arthritis such as rheumatoid or systemic lupus. Greater than 50 000 WBCs with a significant increase in polymorphonuclear cells is highly suggestive of infectious arthritis.

Crystal examination should be performed looking for the strongly negatively birefringent crystals of uric acid and the weakly positive birefringence of calcium pyrophosphate deposition disease. Rarely, cholesterol crystals or glucocorticoid fragments from previous joint injection may be seen in joint fluid.

Injection of a long-acting corticosteroid such as triamcinolone can be effective treatment for an acute joint flare that is not infectious in etiology. A mixture of 1:1 corticosteroid/lidocaine solution can provide acute relief by the lidocaine and a long-term response of up to 3 months by the corticosteroid injection. No more than two to three injections per joint per year are recommended. The need for more frequent injections suggests that an alternative form of therapy might be more appropriate. A series of injections with hyaluronic acid may provide benefit in occasional patients with OA of the hip and knee.

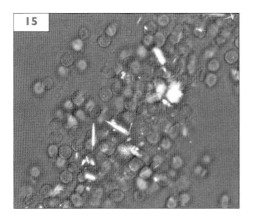

15

15 Synovial fluid analysis under polarized microscopy (dark field examination) reveals multiple birefringent crystals; further examination using red compensator will help to distinguish positive and negative birefringence.

IMAGING

Plain radiographs of the joints can document joint involvement and identify progression of the disease process (**16**). Computed tomography (CT) provides sharper detail and allows cross-sectional imaging (**17**). Magnetic resonance imaging (MRI) is helpful to identify soft tissue disease and has been particularly valuable in rheumatology by imaging the synovium or better defining erosive disease (**18**). Musculoskeletal ultrasound (US) is rapidly growing in popularity and may also be helpful for soft tissue imaging with potential advantages including: 1) lack of radiation exposure (similar to MRI); 2) relative low cost; and 3) adaptability to the clinic setting. Radionuclide scintigraphy may be helpful in demonstrating the extent of arthritis but is very nonspecific and has little application. Likewise, positron emission tomography (PET) scanning is minimally helpful in evaluating painful joints. Classic plain film findings are described in the appropriate chapter.

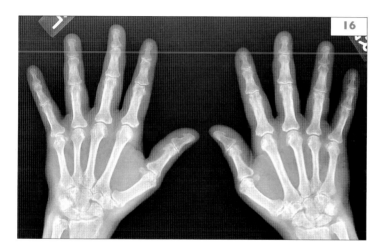

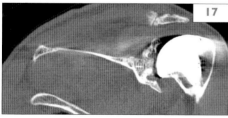

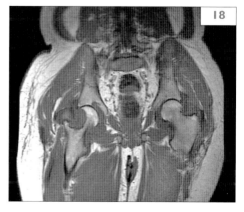

16–18 Imaging modalities commonly used in the evaluation of joint disease. **16**: Radiography in a patient with rheumatoid arthritis; **17**: CT scan in a patient with prior shoulder arthroplasty; **18**: MRI in a patient with amyloidosis.

Pregnancy in rheumatic diseases

INTRODUCTION

There are many treatment and management issues to consider in patients with rheumatic disease, all of which become more complicated in the patient desiring pregnancy. These issues include prepregnancy planning, fertility concerns, fetal and neonatal concerns, medication choices in men and women desiring pregnancy, postpartum care and breast feeding. These issues will be discussed in relation to RA, SLE and related conditions, and systemic sclerosis (scleroderma, SSc).

RHEUMATOID ARTHRITIS

RA is a fairly common disorder that affects women more than men. Many women with RA are of childbearing age, which emphasizes the importance of being prepared for pregnancy. In many patients with RA, disease activity lessens during pregnancy and in the postpartum period. This clinical improvement generally begins in the first trimester and continues well after delivery, although disease flares may occur in the postpartum period. Pregnancy outcomes are generally not impacted by RA; however, medications used can certainly impact fetal development and delivery.

Generally, all women should take requested nutritional supplements, especially folic acid. Smoking, which is associated with increased disease severity in RA, is also discouraged. All medications (including all prescribed and over-the-counter agents) need to be discussed with healthcare providers, with a plan in place in the case of an unplanned pregnancy.

Women on methotrexate (MTX) (a known teratogen) should stop the medication at least 1 month before trying to conceive. In men, 3–4 months is preferable to allow for the development of sperm while free of medication. Women on leflunomide must stop the medication for years prior to pregnancy, unless drug levels are checked and an elimination procedure (using cholestyramine), when appropriate, is used. Other drugs to avoid during pregnancy are cyclophosphamide (CTX) and mycophenolate mofetil (MMF). Biologic medications, including the antitumor necrosis factor (anti-TNF) medications (such as etanercept, infliximab,

adalimumab), anakinra, abatacept, and rituximab should also be avoided due to the lack of information concerning pregnancy and these agents. These medications should also be avoided in the breast-feeding period.

General points to consider include the following:

- Nonsteroidal anti-inflammatory drugs (NSAIDs) cross the placenta and can cause problems during the third trimester of pregnancy, including delayed closure of the patent ductus arteriosus and bleeding complications. NSAIDs should also be avoided in women with fertility issues. A safe alternative during pregnancy is acetaminophen. NSAIDS, with the exception of aspirin, may be used by breast-feeding patients.
- Prednisone is commonly used during pregnancy and is generally felt to be safe. Prednisone crosses the placenta but is seen in small amounts in the developing infant's blood. There have been rare associations of corticosteroid therapy with cleft palates and premature rupture of membranes. Prednisone, preferably in low doses, may be used in the breast-feeding period.
- Azathioprine (AZA) is generally limited to patients with severe RA and extra-articular manifestations. There are conflicting data on its safety, but it is generally felt to be of minimal risk. If AZA is being used for severe extra-articular manifestations such as vasculitis, it may be applicable continue its use during pregnancy. Men who take AZA should stop the medication 3–4 months before their partner tries to conceive due to associations with low sperm counts.
- Sulfasalazine (SSZ) is felt to be of low risk for the developing baby. Most experts agree that it may be continued during pregnancy, though folic acid supplementation of at least 1000 μg per day has been advocated by some clinicians. SSZ is felt to be safe while breast feeding. SSZ can cause reversible male infertility and should be discontinued for 3–4 months prior to conception attempts.
- Hydroxychloroquine (HCQ) is felt to be safe in pregnancy and breast feeding. As in other autoimmune diseases, HCQ often improves disease outcomes.

Though RA often remains in remission into the postpartum period, patients often flare weeks to months after delivery. In some patients, their first manifestation of RA may be in the postpartum period. It is unclear if breast feeding accelerates the time to this flare. It is advisable to restart DMARDs as soon as possible in the postpartum period.

SYSTEMIC LUPUS ERYTHEMATOSUS

SLE is an autoimmune disease that is most common in young women of childbearing age. Although patients with SLE generally have normal fertility, they do have more pregnancy-related complications. Unlike RA, SLE does not improve during pregnancy, and may actually worsen or flare. Additionally, the manifestations of SLE that require treatment may be life- or organ-threatening, and thus, require treatment in the pregnant female. The outcome for both mother and baby is best when SLE manifestations are controlled for at least 6 months prior to conception.

Pregnancy-related complications are more common is SLE. These complications include:
- Hypertension.
- Preterm delivery.
- Unplanned cesarean sections.
- Postpartum hemorrhage.
- Venous thrombosis.
- Low birth weight.
- Fetal loss.
- Premature delivery.

Pre-eclampsia is more common in SLE patients, especially those with kidney disease or antiphospholipid antibodies (aPLs). Many of the manifestations of pre-eclampsia are confused with SLE flares. The treatment for pre-eclampsia is to deliver the baby, and it may not be until that time when the difference between these two diseases can start to be differentiated.

Women with lupus nephritis have a much higher incidence of pregnancy loss. Many patients will experience a worsening of their renal function, worsening hypertension, and worsening proteinuria.

Neonatal lupus is of particular concern in newborns of patients with SLE who have SSA/Ro and/or SSB/La antibodies. These antibodies can cross the placenta to the developing infant. Neonatal lupus may also occur in neonates from mothers who do not have lupus, but who are positive for the SSA and/or SSB autoantibodies. Neonatal lupus occurs in approximately 2% of all mothers with these antibodies and is typically manifested by:
- Rash which is red and raised and resolves by 6–8 months.
- Serositis.
- Heart block (often irreversible) in the neonate.

The most serious complication of heart block can lead to fetal demise. Mothers with SSA/Ro or SSB/La antibodies should be seen by an obstetrician experienced in high-risk pregnancy, and should be monitored with serial fetal cardiac ultrasounds starting early in pregnancy. Infants with neonatal congenital heart block can be treated with corticosteroids and cardiac pacing. If a mother has had one child with neonatal lupus, her risk of having another affected child is approximately 17%.

As with other pregnant women, all patients should be taking nutritional supplements such as folic acid. The recommendations for medications are the same as those for RA (see above). Medications generally felt to be safe in the pregnant female with SLE are NSAIDs, prednisone, HCQ, and AZA. As previously noted, men who are taking MTX, AZA, MMF, or CTX should stop these medications, if possible, 3–4 months prior to conception attempts. This will allow time for the development of sperm not exposed to the drugs. Women taking MMF and CTX should stop the medication 1 month prior to conception to allow time for drug clearance.

The pregnant woman with antiphospholipid antibody syndrome (APS) cannot take warfarin. These patients may be treated with heparin or low-molecular weight heparin. Chronic heparin administration is associated with accelerated osteoporosis, so these patients need to be on adequate calcium and vitamin D therapy.

In the postpartum period, drug therapy recommendations are similar to RA. Drugs felt to be safe in the breast-feeding patient with SLE are:
- Prednisone.
- HCQ.
- Warfarin (Coumadin).
- NSAIDs, excluding aspirin.

AZA, MTX, and CTX should be avoided in the breast-feeding patient.

Birth control in the patient with lupus may take many forms, including abstinence, barrier methods, and pharmacotherapy. It is important to discuss birth control with SLE patients. Birth control with medications that contain low-dose estrogen (less than 35 µg of ethinyl) is safe for most women, except those with antiphospholipid antibodies or migraines. Progesterone preparations may be appropriate in this group of patients.

SYSTEMIC SCLEROSIS (SSc)

It is general felt that patients with SSc have normal fertility, but like SLE, have a higher rate of pregnancy-related complications, such as spontaneous miscarriage. It is unclear if SSc manifestations worsen during pregnancy, though there seems to be a higher rate of renal crisis. This is further complicated by the fact that angiotensin-converting enzyme (ACE) inhibitors, used to treat and prevent renal crisis in SSc, are contraindicated in pregnancy. Another consideration is patients with pulmonary hypertension since there is a high mortality in pregnant woman with pulmonary hypertension. It may be argued that screening for pulmonary hypertension is wise in the patient with SSc contemplating pregnancy. Other manifestations of SSc that may be exacerbated during pregnancy are shortness of breath in the patient with interstitial lung disease, and dyspepsia in the patient with esophageal dysmotility.

Pharmacological treatment of rheumatic disease

INTRODUCTION

Recent decades have dramatically advanced the ability to manage inflammatory rheumatic disease pharmacologically. A paradigm shift from aggressive therapy only once joint destruction has occurred, to early and aggressive therapy to prevent joint destruction, and in some cases induce remission, has served patients well. Unfortunately, remittive agents for noninflammatory arthritis are not yet available, and pain management coupled with nonpharmacological therapy is utilized. The following chapter outlines commonly used agents in rheumatology.

NONSTEROIDAL ANTI-INFLAMMATORY DRUGS

NSAIDs block the synthesis of prostaglandins (PGs), accounting for their anti-inflammatory and analgesic properties. They are widely used as adjunctive therapy in many rheumatic diseases. All NSAIDs block cyclo-oxygenase- (COX) 1 and 2, the precursor for PG synthesis, at variable levels. NSAIDs which selectively block COX-2, may have fewer gastrointestinal complications, but both may be associated with an increased incidence of cardiovascular disease. Risk factors must be assessed before use of NSAIDs in individual patients. Individuals remaining on long-term NSAIDs need to have periodic blood pressure and kidney and liver function monitoring.

There is no difference in efficacy between each NSAID; however, the individual patient may have very different results. It is reasonable to give a 2-week trial of an NSAID and if no results are seen, change to a separate class of NSAID.

GLUCOCORTICOIDS

Glucocorticoids (GCs) are widely used to treat rheumatic disease. The GCs vary widely in their dosage, potency, biologic half-life and mineralicorticoid effects. They can be administered orally, parenterally, intramuscularly and intraarticularly. GCs are anti-inflammatory by direct down-regulation of the immune response of T cells and macrophages. They have little direct effect on B cells or neutrophils, though they do inhibit the adhesion of neutrophils to endothelial cells. The end result is an overall increase in leukocytes, primarily from neutrophils, and a decrease in lymphocytes.

GCs are very effective immunosuppressant drugs and have disease-modifying properties. Unfortunately, they have a myriad of side-effects. Adrenal suppression can occur with low-dose and short-term administration (7.5 mg of predniso-lone for at least 3 weeks). Individuals should be cautioned about this and guidelines given for illness or procedures that may increase physiologic stress. Some patients develop prominent physical changes, which include weight gain, moon facies, striae (**19**), hirsutism, and a buffalo hump. Vigilance for and protection from more serious side-effects is warranted, including osteoporosis, osteonecrosis (**20**), diabetes, dyslipidemia, atherosclerosis, hypertension, myopathy, cataracts, glaucoma, and mood disturbance. Every effort should be made to minimize the dosage and duration of GC usage. High-dose GCs (1–2 mg/kg/day) are frequently indicated in the treatment of systemic vasculitis, polymyositis, and end-organ involvement in SLE. In contrast, much lower doses (5–10 mg/day of prednisone) may be highly effective in the treatment of synovitis related to RA.

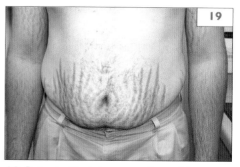

19 Patient with violaceous striae on his abdomen and axilla/upper arms from chronic glucocorticoid use.

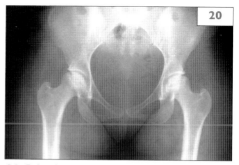

20 Pelvic X-ray showing bilateral osteonecrosis (avascular necrosis) of the femoral heads from glucocorticoid use.

DISEASE MODIFYING ANTIRHEUMATIC DRUGS (DMARDS) AND IMMUNOREGULATORY DRUGS

DMARDs and immunoregulatory drugs are a 'class' of rheumatic drugs that exert immunobiologic effects and were developed out of a need to reduce or spare individuals from GC use. They include antimicrobials, chemotherapeutics, and drugs synthesized directly for rheumatic diseases. A lengthy discussion of the mechanism of action of each of these agents is beyond the scope of this textbook. Many of these agents are used in combination. A list of the most commonly used agents, their general indications, monitoring parameters, and effects on pregnancy and lactation is shown in *Table 3*. Several of these agents have notable drug interactions. HCQ may potentiate hypoglycemia in patients on oral diabetes medications. MTX should be used with caution with other drugs that are known hepatotoxins. Trimethaprim–sulfamethoxazole may decrease MTX clearance and result in hematologic toxicity. NSAIDs and aspirin may also increase levels of MTX, but are often used in combination and require monitoring with changes in dosage. Leflunomide levels are reduced with concomitant cholestyramine administration. Allopurinol (a urate-lowering drug used in gout) also inhibits xanthine oxidase and may result in fatal agranulocytosis when used in combination with AZA. Cyclosporine has many drug interactions, including certain antibiotics, statins, and calcium channel blockers. A complete review of concomitant medication use should be done prior to initiation of cyclosporine. CTX levels are increased by both allopurinol and cimetidine.

Table 3 Disease-modifying, antirheumatic drugs and immunoregulatory drugs used in the treatment of rheumatic conditions

Name	Indications	Monitoring	Side-effects	Pregnancy/lactation
Hydroxychloroquine 200–400 mg/day (not to exceed 6.5 mg/kg/day)	RA, SLE, JIA, APS, MCTD, Sjögren's syndrome	No routine lab monitoring; regular eye examinations	Retinopathy, neuromyopathy Lowers blood glucose	Relatively safe in pregnancy and lactation
Sulfasalazine 1500–3000 mg/day	RA, JIA, arthritis of AS, PsA, ReA	CBC in 2 weeks CBC/ALT/Cr q mo × 3 then q 3 mo	Cytopenia, headache, rash, nausea/diarrhea	Reversible oligospermia Relatively safe in pregnancy and lactation
Methotrexate 7.5–25 mg/week PO, SC, or IM	RA, JIA, SLE, myositis, vasculitis, PsA	CBC/ALT/Cr/Alb q mo × 3 then q 3 mo Baseline: HBV and HCV status and chest X-ray Vaccinations should be up to date	Cytopenia, hepatotoxicity, nausea, stomatitis, alopecia, pneumonitis, methotrexate flu	Discontinue for 3 months before conception (men and women) Category X for pregnancy, not safe in lactation
Leflunomide 10–20 mg/day	RA, SLE, PsA	CBC/ALT/Cr/Alb q mo × 3 then q 3 mo	Hepatotoxicity, diarrhea, weight loss	Check levels prior to conception Category X for pregnancy, not safe in lactation*
Tetracyclines: minocycline 100 mg bid doxycycline 100 mg bid	RA, OA	Periodic liver function tests	Dizziness, nausea, photosensitization, minocycline: hyperpigmentation (**21, 22**), drug-induced lupus	Contraindicated in both

Name	Indications	Monitoring	Side-effects	Pregnancy/lactation
Azathioprine 1–2.5 mg/kg/day	SLE, RA, myositis, vasculitis	May check TPMT genotype, CBC q 2 wk, then monthly, LFTs q 3 mo	Myelosuppression, hypersensitivity, pancreatitis	Relatively safe in pregnancy, caution with lactation
Mycophenylate mofetil 1500–3000 mg/day	SLE, RA, myositis, vasculitis	CBC/LFTs q mo × 3, then q 2–3 mo	Nausea, diarrhea, leukopenia, hepatotoxicity	Category X for pregnancy, not safe in lactation
Cyclosporine 2.5–4 mg/kg/day	PsA, SLE, RA	BP/Cr q 2 wk	Hypertension, nephrotoxicity, malignancy, increased hair growth	Not recommended for either
Cyclophosphamide Oral: 2 mg/kg/day IV: 0.5–0.75 mg/m^2/month	SLE nephritis, vasculitis	CBC q 1–2 wk, then q mo	Myelosuppression, hemorrhagic cystitis, bladder and other cancers, sterility, infection	Category X for pregnancy, not safe in lactation

Al: albumin; ALT: alanine aminotransferase; APS: antiphospholipid antibody syndrome; AS: ankylosing spondylitis; BP: blood pressure; CBC: complete blood count; Cr: creatine; HBV: hepatitis B virus; HCV: hepatitis C virus; JIA: juvenile idiopathic arthritis; LFT: liver function test; MCTD: mixed connective tissue disease; OA: osteoarthritis; PsA: psoriatic arthritis; RA: rheumatoid arthritis; ReA: reactive arthritis; SLE: systemic lupus erythematosus; TPMT: thiopurine S-methyltransferase; UA: urinalysis.

* Leflunomide has a long half-life due (up to 6 weeks or longer) and levels may remain elevated for lengthy periods following drug discontinuation; a 'washout' with cholestyramine should be considered if levels are elevated.

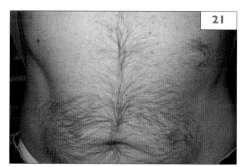

21 Patient with minocycline hyperpigmentation at the sites of his insulin injections.

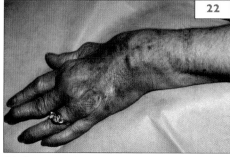

22 Patient with hyperpigmentation from minocycline therapy for her rheumatoid arthritis.

BIOLOGIC AGENTS

More recently, agents used in rheumatic disease target specific aspects of the immune response, such as cytokines and cellular molecules. They are collectively referred to as the biologic agents (*Table 4*).

TNF-α plays a central role in many inflammatory conditions. Current strategies to block TNF-α include monoclonal antibodies or soluble receptors to TNF-α, which bind to and render TNF-α inactive. IL-1 is also fundamental in the inflammatory response, and the currently available agent, which blocks IL-1, involves competitive inhibition by a homologue of the native receptor. In addition to targeting cytokines, agents that target B cells via the CD20 membrane receptor and agents that target T cells by inhibition of CD80 and CD86 co-stimulation are

Table 4 Biologic agents used in the treatment of rheumatic diseases

Name	Mechanism of action	Indications

Infliximab
  3 mg/kg IV with load
  then q 8 wk
	Chimeric monoclonal
	  Ab against TNF-α
		RA, PsA, AS

Etanercept
  50 mg q wk SC
	TNF-α receptor
	  fused to human IgG1
		RA, PsA, AS

Adalimumab
  40 mg q 2 wk
	Humanized
	  monoclonal Ab against TNF-α
		RA, PsA, AS

Golimumab
  50 mg q mo SC
	Humanized
	  monoclonal Ab against TNF-α
		RA, PsA, AS

Certolizumab
  400 mg SC weeks
  0, 2, 4 then 200 mg
  q 2 wk
	Humanized monoclonal Ab
	  against TNF-α (Fab region only);
	  PEG conjugated
		RA

Tocilizumab
  4–8 mg/kg IV q 4 wk
	Humanized monoclonal
	  Ab against IL-6 receptor
		RA

Anakinra
  100 mg qd SC
	Recombinant IL-1
	  receptor antagonist
		RA, auto-inflammatory
		  diseases

Rituximab
  1000 mg IV day
  1 and 15
	Monoclonal Ab
	  against CD20 on B cells
		RA, possibly
		  SLE, APS

Abatacept
  10 mg/kg IV q mo
	Fusion protein of CTLA-4 and
	  IgG1 that binds CD80 and CD86
	  and blocks T cell activation
		RA

Ab: antibody; APS: antiphospholipid antibody syndrome; AS: ankylosing spondylitis; Ig: immunoglobulin; IL: interleukin; PEG: polyethylene glycol; PsA: psoriatic arthritis; RA: rheumatoid arthritis; SLE: systemic lupus erythematosus; TNF: tumor necrosis factor.

available. There are numerous additional biologic agents in development.

All of these agents increase the risk of infection. Individuals should be screened for TB and hepatitis B prior to initiation of treatment. Vigilance should be maintained for any signs or symptoms of all infections, while taking these very potent immunosuppressant agents. Anti-TNF agents have been associated with an increased incidence of serious infection including systemic fungal infections and TB. All patients should be screened for latent TB prior to their initiation. In general, biologic agents are routinely used in combination with DMARDs and immuno-regulatory drugs, but should not be used in combination with each other.

COLCHICINE

Colchicine is a tubular toxin that inhibits neutrophil motility. It is effective in the treatment of acute gout (daily oral doses of 0.6 mg bid to tid) and in the prevention of gout flares, particularly with the initiation of urate-lowering medicines. Although available as an IV preparation, great caution should be used with this dosing route given the very narrow therapeutic index associated with IV administration. Gastrointestinal side-effects (nausea and diarrhea) are dose dependent. Colchicine is also used to treat pseudogout (calcium pyrophosphate dehydrate, CPPD), familial Mediterranean fever (FMF), and inflammatory pericarditis.

URATE-LOWERING MEDICATIONS

Allopurinol is a potent xanthine oxidase inhibitor, the rate limiting enzyme in uric acid synthesis. It is effective in lowering serum urate levels and reducing (even eliminating) gout flares. Allopurinol is effective in underexcreters (~80% of gout patients) and overproducers and is approved for a daily dose up to 800 mg. Initial allopurinol dosing should be adjusted for renal impairment and strong consideration should be given to anti-inflammatory prophylaxis (colchicine or NSAIDs) to prevent rebound gout flares. Rarely, patients can develop allopurinol hypersensitivity which can be severe. Febuxostat (Uloric) is also a xanthine oxidase inhibitor approved for the treatment of gout. In general, allopurinol is still the treatment of choice. Probenecid is an uricouric agent and can be useful in the treatment of chronic gout. It is effective in underexcretors but not overproducers, is not effective in the context of renal impairment

(glomerular filtration rate [GFR] <50 ml/min) and should be used with caution in patients with a history of nephrolithiasis.

MISCELLANEOUS AGENTS

Acetaminophen (paracetamol) is commonly used in rheumatic disease. It is strictly analgesic and not anti-inflammatory. This suggests that its effects are primarily limited to the central nervous system where it may exert its influence via COX-3. While acetaminophen is generally regarded as safe in dosages up to 4000 mg daily, the lowest effective dosage should be determined and maintained. Acetaminophen is present in many prescriptions and over-the-counter medications and patients should be counseled not to exceed the safe daily dosage.

Glucosamine and chondroitin sulfate, at dosages of 1500 mg/day and 1200 mg/day have been used with some success in OA, although more recent evidence has suggested minimal to no benefit.

PEARLS

- Physical therapy and nonpharmacological modalities should not be forgotten! Patients on even short-term and low-dose GCs may develop adrenal insufficiency and should be educated that increases in physiologic stress require an increase in their dosage. Concomitant use of AZA and allopurinol may result in fatal agranulocytosis. The dose of AZA must be reduced if allopurinol is to be used.
- Patients should be checked for both TB and hepatitis B prior to initiating biologic agents.
- DMARDS, immunoregulatory, and biologic agents should be used when appropriate to reduce GC use.

Nonpharmacological treatment of rheumatic disease

INTRODUCTION

There are several nonpharmacologic treatments for rheumatic diseases, and these should not be overlooked. Co-ordinated care with a physical therapist, occupational therapist, orthotist, and nutritionist can lead to significant functional improvements and reduce morbidity from arthritis. Referral to a therapist can seem confusing when the primary care practitioner is not familiar with all of the possible therapies, devices, and modalities available. It is within the scope of the therapists' practice to determine the most effective modality and parameters for treatment. If a referral is appropriate, one solution is to write the referral with the diagnosis listed and the following: 'evaluate and treat', with specific additional instructions if so desired. This allows the therapist to develop an appropriate treatment plan.

ASSISTIVE DEVICES

Patients with arthritis in the lower extremity frequently present with pain during weight bearing activities. These individuals, especially those with hip or knee OA, may benefit from unloading, or decreased weight bearing, on the lower extremity. Assistive devices, such as canes or walkers, allow unloading of one or both lower extremities to decrease pain as well as compensate for muscle weakness or provide stability for balance deficits. Assistive devices with a broader base of support offer more stability, but slow gait speed and hinder environmental accessibility.

However, wheels are available for quad canes and walkers to maximize stability, yet minimize limitation in gait speed. When prescribing an assistive device for a patient with arthritis, co-morbid conditions, lifestyle, and living arrangements should be considered. Referral to a physical therapist for device prescription is indicated when an individual has significant health limitations, balance deficits, and/or gait deviations.

Many patients with lower extremity arthritis ambulate easily under normal circumstances, but have difficulty in challenging situations such as walking longer distances, on uneven terrain, or during adverse weather conditions. Use of an assistive device under these conditions can prevent torques and shear forces across degenerated joint surfaces from reaching harmful levels and exacerbating signs and symptoms of arthritis. Recommending that the patient have a cane or retractable walking stick (**23**) available during these circumstances can protect the joint and enhance safety. For regular cane users, addition of a tripod or ice pick tip in the winter will increase sense of security (**24, 25**).

For assistive devices to be effective they need to be utilized correctly. Devices should be fit so that the handgrip is at the level of the ulnar styloid and the elbow is in approximately 15° of flexion. A cane or single crutch should be used on the side **opposite** the affected lower extremity. For all devices, when ambulating on level surfaces, the assistive device should be advanced with the affected lower extremity during the gait cycle. When ascending stairs, the unaffected lower extremity should lead, followed by the affected lower extremity and assistive device. If descending, the pattern is reversed; the assistive device and affected lower extremity are lowered to the step below, followed by the unaffected extremity. If a patient is nonweight bearing the sequence for level and stair ambulation is the same, except that the involved limb does not touch the ground.

PHYSICAL AGENTS/TREATMENT MODALITIES

Joint and tissue dysfunction of various etiologies may be treated with application of a physical agent. These modalities use the physical properties of heat, electricity, or sound to alter tissue inflammation and promote healing. The tissue injured, tissue depth, and size of involved area determine which physical agent will be effective in managing a given condition. *Table 5* describes several modalities, their indications, and contraindications. If a physical agent may be helpful, a general referral to a physical or occupational therapist is appropriate.

PHYSICAL ACTIVITY PRESCRIPTION

Physical activity and exercise has consistently been demonstrated to be safe and beneficial for individuals with OA as well as those with

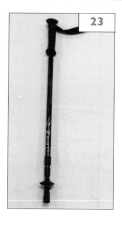

23 Retractable walking stick.

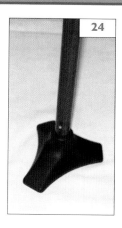

24 Cane tip adaptations: tripod.

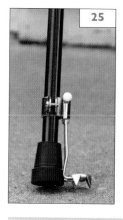

25 Cane tip adaptations: ice pick.

Table 5 Physical agents/treatment modalities

Physical agent	Description/indications	Contraindications
Cold packs	Use: Superficial application of cold is effective to control acute inflammation, edema and temporarily decrease pain Indications: Acute injury, postsurgery, arthritis joint pain	Raynaud's syndrome Over a regenerating nerve Impaired circulation
Hot packs	Use: Superficial application of heat has a depth of penetration of ~0.5 cm. Use for pain control and to decrease tissue stiffness. Evidence for effectiveness is minimal; the effect is small and temporary Indications: Muscle spasms secondary to low back pain, tissue stiffness secondary to arthritis	Impaired sensation Impaired cognition Potential for hemorrhage Precautions: Acute tissue injury Pregnancy Impaired circulation Edema

(continued)

Table 5 Physical agents/treatment modalities (continued)

Physical agent	Description/indications	Contraindications
Ultrasound (US)		
Thermal (continuous) US	Use: The US waveform is applied continuously and penetrates to a depth of 2–5 cm. The thermal effects cause increased tissue extensibility to increase muscle length or joint ROM. Thought to decrease pain and increase healing, although the evidence is not strong Indications: Joints painful secondary to OA, but not swollen.	Malignancy Pregnancy Prosthetic joint cement Over plastic prosthetic components Thrombophlebitis Precautions: Epiphyseal plates Fractures
Nonthermal (pulsed) US	Use: US waveform is applied in intermittent bursts (pulses). Tissue temperature does not elevate, but mechanical effects are anti-inflammatory and promote tissue healing at depths of up to 5 cm Indications: Inflamed joints and joint related structures, soft tissue injury. Can also deliver medication (dexamethasone or ketoprofen) via phonophoresis	
Electrical stimulation (ES)	There are multiple applications for ES as described below.	
Transcutaneous electrical nerve stimulation (TENS)	Use: Electric current stimulates the sensory nerve fibers to block the pain pathways which carry pain messages to the brain Indications: Chronic pain, postsurgical pain	For all electrical modalities: Cardiac pacemaker Placement over the carotid sinuses
Neuromuscular ES (NMES)	Use: Intermittent electrical current is used at an intensity to depolarize the motor nerve which stimulates a muscle contraction. This is used to strengthen or re-educate weak muscles or reduce muscle spasm Indications: Used as a modality for muscle strengthening or re-education of the quadriceps in cases of severe knee arthritis or post surgery Application for reduction of muscle spasms associated with low back pain is also a common There is more evidence for use of NMES for muscle strengthening, but less for remediation of muscle spasms	Thrombophlebitis Precautions: Pregnancy Tumor Poor tolerance due to discomfort Areas of skin irritation
Iontophoresis	Use: Application of anti-inflammatory (dexamethasone) or pain control medication via electric current Indications: Used to address localized areas of inflammation; effective for tendonitis in superficial areas such as the supraspinatus, lateral epicondylitis, and patellar tendonitis.	

ES: electrical stimulation; NMES: neuromuscular electrical stimulation; OA: osteoarthritis; ROM: range of motion; TENS: transcutaneous electrical nerve stimulation.

inflammatory types of arthritis. In addition to the general health benefit of physical activity programs, persons with arthritis often experience a decrease in pain and improved function. The US Department of Health and Human Services and CDC 2008 Guidelines for Physical Activity recommend both aerobic and resistance training for adults. The guidelines recommend a total weekly accumulation of 150 minutes of moderate physical activity and 2–3 sessions of resistance training for all major muscle groups. This dose of physical activity is recommended for persons with arthritis as well as healthy adults because similar programs have been demonstrated to be safe and effective for persons with arthritis without negative consequences to the diseased joint. In addition to these general recommendations, quadriceps strengthening is suggested for persons with knee arthritis. Individuals with anterior knee pain or patellofemoral arthritis are most likely to benefit from this type of exercise.

Most persons with arthritis who exercise or participate in physical activity programs will experience improvement; however, there can be a temporary increase in pain during the first weeks after initiating activity. To minimize joint pain and inflammation, exercise intensity and duration should be increased incrementally. Activity should be modified if discomfort becomes pain during exercise or continues for an extended period after exercise has ended. If exercise is tolerated poorly, the activity can be performed in small bouts rather than as a single session, or exercise can be performed in water to minimize weight bearing. During symptomatic periods, patients should decrease activity to a tolerable level, but not stop, as discontinuation of activity will result in a rapid and significant loss of functional capacity. Exercise specialists at community health centers can assist persons with arthritis to design a general fitness program. Referral to a physical therapist for exercise is indicated for persons with one or more of the following complications:

- Severe OA of a weight-bearing joint.
- Complications from arthritis that require modification of standard exercises.
- Multiple co-morbid conditions putting an individual at high risk for exercise.
- Joint dysfunction requiring specific exercise prescription.
- Prior adverse response to exercise.

MECHANICAL BRACING

Braces mechanically realign joints with arthritis normalizing biomechanics. Avoidance of harmful movement results in improved function and decreased pain. *Table 6 overleaf* describes some available devices.

JOINT RANGE OF MOTION (ROM)/MANUAL THERAPY

Evidence-based practice guidelines recommend joint ROM exercise in a comprehensive arthritis management program. Manual therapy refers to the manual techniques performed by a physical therapist to address joint capsule adhesions and ROM limitations, with the goal to maintain or restore motion of joints with arthritis. For patients with OA of the hip or lumbar spinal stenosis, recent research suggests manual therapy may be an efficacious, noninvasive intervention to decrease pain and restore function.

WEIGHT LOSS

A high body mass index (BMI) is associated with an increased incidence of knee OA. Weight loss is an effective intervention to decrease pain and disability secondary to the disease. As other co-morbid conditions, such as hypertension and diabetes, are associated with obesity, weight loss may also lead to improvements in overall health. Motivated individuals who have not had weight-loss success with prior attempts at dieting, or who have other chronic diseases exacerbated by obesity, may benefit from referral to a medical nutrition professional.

Table 6 Devices for mechanical bracing of joints

Device	Description
Ring splints (**26**; Courtesy of www.silverringsplint.com.)	Treats and prevents finger deformities in individuals with inflammatory types of arthritis Occupational therapists can recommend and fit the appropriate splint
Unloader braces (**27**; Courtesy of www.donjoy.com.)	Indicated for unicompartmental OA of the knee; brace allows a unidirectional force to be applied to decrease varus or valgus forces Brace should be worn during weight-bearing activities Unloader braces can be fitted by and purchased from an orthotist
Wedges (**28**; Courtesy of www.feetrelief.com.)	In cases of unicompartmental knee OA, medial or lateral wedges are inserted into the shoe, used to alter lower extremity joint biomechanics, decreasing varus or valgus force at the knee
Orthotic shoe inserts (**29**)	Prefabricated or custom inserts for shoes support the foot and distribute weight bearing throughout the plantar surface of the foot, indicated for persons with OA of any area of the foot or ankle as in normal biomechanics Orthotics are also effective in the prevention and treatment of plantar fasciitis as they minimize pronation

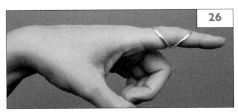

26 Ring splint; treats and prevents finger deformities in inflammatory types of arthritis.

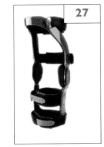

27 Unloader brace for unicompartmental osteoarthritis of the knee; brace allows a unidirectional force to be applied to decrease varus or valgus forces.

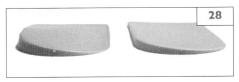

28 Medial or lateral wedges are inserted into the shoe for use in unicompartmental knee osteoarthritis; used to alter lower extremity joint biomechanics, decreasing varus or valgus force at the knee.

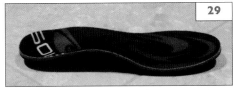

29 Orthotic shoe insert used to support the foot and distribute weight bearing throughout the plantar surface of the foot to promote normal biomechanics and minimize pronation; indicated for osteoarthritis of any area of the foot or ankle and in the prevention and treatment of plantar fasciitis.

Osteoarthritis and Inflammatory Arthritis

- **Osteoarthritis**
- **Rheumatoid arthritis**
- **Gout**
- **CPPD deposition, pseudogout, and chondrocalcinosis**
- **Adult-onset Still's disease**
- **Septic arthritis**
- **Viral arthritis**
- **Lyme disease**
- **Rheumatic fever**

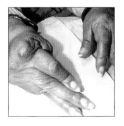
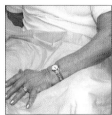
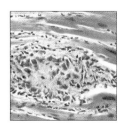
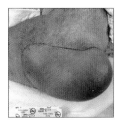

Osteoarthritis

DEFINITION

Osteoarthritis (OA) is a slowly progressive form of arthritis, the product of cartilage failure resulting in progressive joint space narrowing, bony proliferation, and pain. Other common names for OA include osteoarthrosis and degenerative joint disease (DJD).

EPIDEMIOLOGY AND ETIOLOGY

OA is strongly age-related and is uncommon before the age of 40 years. Prevalence increases with age and is nearly universal in individuals over the age of 70 years. It is estimated that ~12% of US adults have clinically relevant OA; the number approaches one in three in elderly populations. OA is the most common indication for total joint replacement surgery, currently one of the most common elective surgeries performed. Important risk factors for OA are:
• Increasing age.
• Female gender (especially in the knees and hands).
• Family history (suggesting a strong genetic component).
• Obesity (especially in OA of the knees).
• Trauma.

OA can develop under normal load circumstances and under excessive load circumstances as seen in trauma. In both cases, as the cartilage fails, excessive forces are placed on the underlying bone.

PATHOGENESIS

OA can be defined as a gradual loss of articular cartilage leading to subchondral bone thickening and subsequent bony outgrowths called osteophytes. These osteophytes are found at the joint margins and may be associated with low-grade inflammation. This process is different from normal aging.

The homeostasis of articular cartilage is controlled by the chondrocyte. OA results from chondrocyte failure. Ultimately what is seen is an imbalance between matrix synthesis and degradation. Abnormalities noted can be described as early and late findings.

Early
• Swelling of the articular cartilage.
• Breakdown of the collagen network responsible for tensile strength and hydrophilia.
• Increased proteoglycan synthesis and release of degradative enzymes, such as matrix metalloproteinases, and aggrecanase, that degrade matrix.

Late
• Degradation enzymes break down proteoglycans faster than they are produced by the chondrocyte.
• The articular cartilage thins and joint space narrowing begins.
• Fissuring and cracking of the cartilage is noted resulting in exposure of the underlying bone.
• Synovial fluid can be forced into adjacent bone resulting in cysts and geodes.
• Hypertrophy of the subchondral bone begins and eventually leads to osteophytes and sclerosis.

Although OA is considered a noninflammatory process, there are inflammatory cytokines that provide signals resulting in chondrocyte-released, cartilage-degrading enzymes. Interleukin (IL)-1 is felt to be the central player in this process, though other cytokines are also important.

CLINICAL HISTORY

The most common features of OA are activity-related pain, minimal morning stiffness (in contrast to inflammatory arthritis), and relatively little joint swelling. One of the interesting features of OA is that joint changes on radiographs and patient-described symptoms are often incongruent.

Although OA can theoretically affect any synovial lined joint in the body, the joints typically affected are:
• Hands: distal and proximal interphalangeal (DIP, PIP) joints and the first carpal–metacarpal (CMC) joint.
• Acromial clavicular joint of the shoulder.
• Cervical and lumbar–sacral spine.
• Hip joint.
• Knee joint.
• In the foot, the first metatarsal–phalangeal (MTP) joint.

Involvement of other joints of the body (atypical joints such as the wrist or elbow) should raise suspicion that there is a secondary cause for the patient's arthritis. Also, it is important to remember that the end result of any inflammatory arthritis is a degenerative joint.

In OA, joints are often involved in an asymmetrical fashion, unlike end-stage inflammatory arthritis. For instance, in the knee, the medial joint space may be involved without associated involvement of the lateral side. This can be a helpful finding when evaluating the etiology of a patient's symptoms.

Though OA clearly represents a spectrum of disease, defining distinct subsets is difficult. OA is associated with trauma, but little can be predicted with respect to the degree of trauma needed and the time frame when symptoms will occur. There is a genetic predisposition, though the penetrance is incomplete. One group that does seem to be unique is erosive OA, or inflammatory OA subset. Typically this is seen in postmenopausal women and is characterized by pain, swelling, and inflammation in the interphalangeal joints of the hands. With time this inflammation subsides and the patient is left with a deformed, and rarely, an ankylosed joint.

Another subset often described is generalized OA, called Kellgren's syndrome. These individuals have typical OA in several joint groups, often more than four. The disease may manifest earlier than usual, in 40–50-year-olds (suggesting a strong genetic component), and X-ray findings may be more severe.

Diffuse idiopathic skeletal hyperostosis (DISH) is a subset of OA that affects the spine and is characterized by bridging osteophytes in the spine resulting from calcification of the anterior longitudinal ligament. Patients may also have enthesophytes and osteophytes of peripheral joints. The typical patient is an older obese male patient with diabetes.

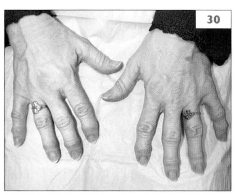

30 Heberden's and Bouchard's nodes are due to bony 'overgrowth' at the distal interphalangeal and proximal interphalangeal joints, respectively. (Dr G F Moore collection)

PHYSICAL EXAMINATION

Clinical features that are present include:

- Joint enlargement. Bouchard's and Heberden's nodes of the PIP and DIP joints, respectively, may be found and a 'shelf sign' of the first CMC joint (**30**).
- Cool effusions in the knees reflecting a 'noninflammatory' process.
- Limitations of joint mobility and crepitus with associated muscle atrophy.

DIFFERENTIAL DIAGNOSIS

Diagnosing OA is not difficult. The difficulty is in ensuring that the degenerative arthritis is typical OA versus atypical OA. There are many causes of secondary OA (*Table 7*). This diagnosis should be entertained in the patient that has degenerative changes in an atypical joint distribution, or the patient has premature degenerative findings. In addition to an atypical joint distribution and precocious onset, another important clue suggesting secondary or atypical OA includes the degree of individual joint involvement (symmetrical versus asymmetrical). An evaluation for metabolic or endocrine disorders is particularly important when assessing for secondary OA.

INVESTIGATIONS

The key to an OA diagnosis is the history and physical, like many other diseases managed by rheumatologists. The role of laboratory testing is minimal. As expected with a noninflammatory process, the erythrocyte sedimentation rate (ESR) and C-reactive protein (CRP) are typically normal. Serological testing, to include rheumatoid factor (RF) and antinuclear antibody (ANA), are also negative.

Joint aspiration typically demonstrates a noninflammatory fluid which is relatively clear and viscous. The total cell count will be less than 2000 cells/mm³ (fewer polymorphonuclear cells [PMNs]) and the microscopic analysis will be free from crystals.

Radiographs are often helpful in evaluation. The bone mineralization is normal to increased. Cartilage spaces will be narrowed, often with asymmetry from one side of the joint to the other (**31**). It is important to complete weight-bearing films in the lower extremities to see the narrowing. Deformities are commonly related to osteophytes, Bouchard's nodes, and Heberden nodes. Erosions are absent, though there is a form of OA called erosive OA. In this variant patient will have 'central erosions' of the PIP and DIP joints of the hands, with characteristic 'gull winging' (**32**). In the back, a collection of nitrogen in a degenerated disc space may be seen, termed a 'vacuum sign'. Changes in the subchondral bone are often found, including cysts, geodes, and sclerosis.

Table 7 Secondary causes of osteoarthritis

Trauma
Inflammatory arthritis
Metabolic disorders

Hemachromatosis
Ochronosis
Gaucher's disease
Sickle cell anemia and other hemaglobinopathies
Magnesium metabolism disorders
Hypophosphatasia

Endocrine disorders

Parathyroid disorders
Thyroid disorders
Acromegaly

Neuropathic joints
Congenital disorders

Legg–Calvé–Perthes
Congenital hip dislocation
Slipped capital femoral epiphysis
Congenital shallow femoral acetabulum
Spondyloepiphyseal dysplasia or congenital dwarfism

HISTOLOGY

Histological changes are dependent on the stage of OA. In early OA, the articular cartilage surface becomes irregular and clefts begin to appear. Histochemical staining demonstrates an alteration in proteoglycan distribution and type I collagen concentrations. As OA progresses, the sub-chondral bone becomes exposed. Eventually, marginal osteophytes form which are covered with hyaline and fibrocartilage. The consequence is abnormal joint homeostasis, altered joint loading mechanics, and increased joint friction from poor lubrication.

PROGNOSIS

There is no uniform prognosis for patients with OA. The prognosis depends on many factors such as involved joints and occupation. Generally, OA is asymptomatic for years while slowly progressing. The rate of progression is variable though seems to be more rapid once symptomatic. OA can lead to severe disability from motion limitations and joint pain.

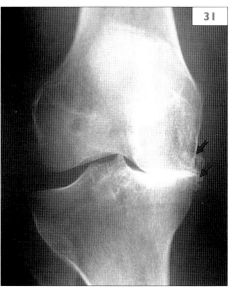

31 Asymmetric joint space narrowing of the medial joint space in knee osteoarthritis with marked osteophyte formation (arrows). (Courtesy Dr GF Moore.)

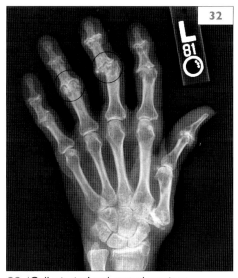

32 'Gull winging' and central erosions (circles) of the interphalangeal joints of the hands related to erosive osteoarthritis. (Courtesy Dr GF Moore.)

MANAGEMENT

The treatment of OA is largely driven by joint symptoms and not radiographic findings. All the therapy to date is to decrease symptoms. No existing therapy impacts disease progression. Investigations continue into potential disease-modifying interventions.

A multifaceted approach is often used with physical and occupational therapy, exercise with muscle strengthening, weight loss, and patient education acting as the foundation. Splints, canes, shoe lateral wedged insoles (for medial compartment knee OA), and other assistive devices are often helpful. Topical therapies include capsaicin, topical nonsteroidal anti-inflammatory drugs (NSAIDs), and lidocaine patches. Systemic therapy includes acetaminophen (paracetamol), NSAIDs, non-acetylated salicylates, and narcotic analgesics.

For patients with more severe disease, other treatments available include joint injection with corticosteroids or, in the knee, hyaluronic acid derivatives. Nutritional supplements such as glucosamine and chondroitin sulfate have been studied in OA and may be modestly beneficial in some patients. Joint replacement, most often performed in the knee and hip, is often very helpful for patients with severe, refractory disease.

Rheumatoid arthritis

DEFINITION

Rheumatoid arthritis (RA) is a systemic autoimmune disease of unknown etiology that primarily targets synovial joints. Synovial tissues proliferate unchecked and result in stretching of tendons and ligaments and bony destruction with resultant deformities and disability.

EPIDEMIOLOGY AND ETIOLOGY

RA is found in up to 1% of adults and is approximately three times more common in women than men. Women have an increasing incidence of RA until approximately age 50 and then the incidence plateaus. Therefore, RA in women of child-bearing age is not rare. RA in men before 40 years of age is uncommon but then steadily increases. New-onset RA is not uncommon in men or women in the seventh to ninth decade.

The cause(s) of RA remains elusive but appears to result from a complex interaction between multiple genes and the environment. Important risk factors include:
• HLA-DR4 shared epitope.
• Smoking.

HLA-DR4 'shared epitope' refers to a common amino acid sequence found in the hypervariable regions of select HLA-DR alleles and is the genetic factor most strongly associated with RA risk. The shared epitope is common, present in approximately 25% of Caucasians, but alone is not enough to cause RA. Multiple other genes including PTPN22, Traf1, Stat4, and GSTM1 also increase the risk of RA. Further, the concordance rate in monozygote twins approaches 15% suggesting a strong genetic component, but also highlighting the role of other factors. Smoking has clearly been demonstrated to be associated with a subset of RA patients who have antibodies to cyclic citrullinated peptide (CCP) and who are shared epitope positive. Since only about one-third of RA patients have a history of smoking, other environmental factors including periodontal disease and exposure to pollutants or silica are thought to play a role.

PATHOGENESIS

Years before clinical symptoms arise, many patients begin to make high levels of antibodies to CCP that are essentially exclusive to RA, while at the same time also making RF which is more nonspecific. The production of these and other autoantibodies requires a complex interaction of antigen-presenting cells (macrophages and dendritic cells), T cells, and B cells. In the RA joint, many cells are involved including those mentioned above, as well as synoviocytes and neutrophils. Proinflammatory cytokines, including tumor necrosis factor (TNF) and IL-1, are found in abundance in affected tissues as are cytokines that are produced by Th17 cells, including IL-23. Th17 cells appear to drive RA both in the synovial tissue and bone where they are important for the erosions through IL-23's role in activating RANK ligand in concert with IL-6.

CLINICAL HISTORY AND PHYSICAL EXAMINATION

RA onset is often characterized by symmetrical polyarthritis primarily affecting the metacarpal–phalangeal (MCP), PIP, and MTP joints, and prolonged morning stiffness of these joint areas (**33**).

Signs and symptoms of RA may be categorized as systemic, articular, and extra-articular.

Systemic

Given its systemic nature, RA may manifest with fatigue, anemia, and occasionally weight loss. Importantly, systemic inflammation damages blood vessels and leads to premature atherosclerosis.

Articular

Often starting in small joints of the hands (PIPs and MCPs) and feet (MTPs), synovitis can spread to any synovial joint in the body. It starts out as soft tissue swelling secondary to effusions, but if these effusions persist, stretching of

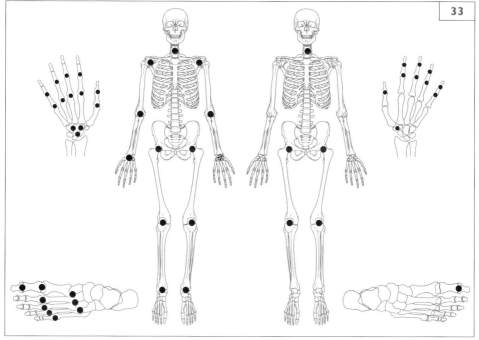

33 Typical joint distributions in rheumatoid arthritis (left) compared with osteoarthritis (right).

tendons and ligaments can lead to deformities (**34–39**). While any synovial joint can be involved, in most patients there is a definite order of involvement from early to late disease:

- Early – MCPs, PIPs, MTPs.
- Intermediate – Wrists, knees, elbows, ankles.
- Late – Hips, shoulders, and C1–C2 articulation.

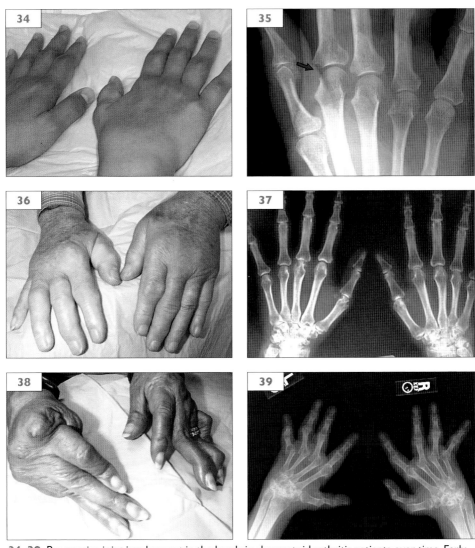

34–39 Progressive joint involvement in the hands in rheumatoid arthritis patients over time. Early findings include symmetrical synovitis in the metacarpal–phalangeal and proximal interphalangeal joints (**34**) along with periarticular osteopenia and early marginal erosions (arrow, **35**). This may progress with persistent synovitis and early palmar subluxation (right hand, **36**) and X-ray changes of more marked osteopenia, joint space narrowing, and progressive erosive changes (**37**). If suboptimally treated this can progress, resulting in marked joint deformities (**38**) and frank destructive changes on X-ray (**39**).

Patients with active RA may develop C1–C2 subluxation (**40**). All clinicians caring for RA patients need to be aware of this, as fatal subluxation can occur if the patient is forced into positions of significant flexion by X-ray technicians or when they are undergoing surgery and under anesthesia.

Extra-articular

- Skin: Subcutaneous nodules are most common (~25%) (**41**); typically they occur in RF positive patients, and are a marker for severe disease. They can also occur in lungs and heart but are most common on the extensor surfaces of elbows.
  - Pyoderma gangrenosum: results in nonhealing skin ulcers, most often affecting the lower extremities.
- Cardiopulmonary sites result in:
  - Coronary artery disease and atherosclerosis.
  - Pleural/pericardial effusions (often asymptomatic); constrictive pericarditis is rare.
  - Interstitial lung disease; bronchiectasis; nodules.
- Sjögren's syndrome can develop. (See section on Sjögren's syndrome, Part 5 Connective Tissue Diseases.)
- Eyes can develop scleritis and episcleritis.
- Hematologic effects include:
  - Anemia of chronic disease.
  - Thrombocytosis – parallels inflammation.
  - Felty's syndrome: triad of leucopenia, splenomegaly, and RA; recurrent infections and leg ulcers.
  - Large granular lymphocyte (LGL) syndrome – marked leucopenia.
- Vasculitis: can be systemic, which may mimic polyarteritis nodosa; or localized vasculitis with subcutaneous nodules and digital infarctions.
- Bone: osteoporosis can develop leading to fracture.

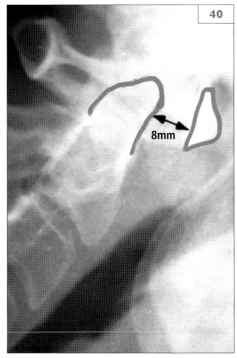

40 Cervical spine radiograph (with forward flexions) showing marked atlanto–axial (C1–C2) subluxation. (Courtesy of Dr GF Moore.)

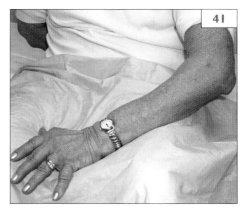

41 Rheumatoid nodules noted over the extensor surface of the elbow in a patient with longstanding rheumatoid arthritis. (Courtesy of Dr GF Moore.)

DIFFERENTIAL DIAGNOSIS

The differential diagnosis of RA is broad. Considerations include viral-associated arthritis (typically self-limited and lasting <6 weeks), OA, and other forms of inflammatory arthritis (i.e. lupus, psoriatic arthritis, or crystalline arthropathy). The distribution of joints involved is often helpful in distinguishing RA from OA (**33**).

Diagnosis of RA remains clinical as evidenced by the disease classification criteria (*Table 8*). Five of the seven 1987 criteria are fulfilled by history or physical examination with only two requiring a laboratory test (RF) or X-rays. Criteria are necessary since no one single test or finding alone can make a diagnosis. To be classified as having RA for study purposes (based on 1987 criteria) ≥four criteria must be met, and the first four criteria must be present for >6 weeks. Given concerns over the lack of sensitivity of these criteria for detecting early disease and the recent recognition of the specificity and early appearance of anticitrullinated peptide antibody (anti-CCP), the RA Classification Criteria have been revised to include anti-CCP positivity (*Table 8*). Well over 90% of patients who present with inflammatory, arthritis-like symptoms and have anti-CCP go on to develop full-blown RA within 3 years.

Table 8 American College of Rheumatology rheumatoid arthritis (RA) classification criteria

1987 Classification criteria – RA present with ≥4 criteria present	2010 Classification criteria (joint initiative with European League against Rheumatism) – RA present if score ≥6 (points)
*Morning stiffness >1 hour	Joint involvement (includes any swollen or tender joint)*
*Arthritis of three joint areas	1 Large joint (0)
*Arthritis of the hands	2–10 large joints (1)
*Symmetrical arthritis	1–3 small joints (2)
Rheumatoid nodules	4–10 small joints (3)
Serum rheumatoid factor	>10 joints (at least 1 small joint) (5)
Typical radiographic changes	
*These criteria must be present for >6 weeks.	Serology†
	Negative RF and negative anti-CCP (0)
	Low positive RF or low positive anti-CCP (2)
	High positive RF or high positive anti-CCP (3)
	Acute phase reactants
	Normal CRP and normal ESR (0)
	Abnormal CRP or abnormal CRP (1)
	Duration of symptoms
	<6 weeks (0)
	≥6 weeks (1)

* Large joints = shoulders, elbows, hips, knees and ankles; small joints = MCP, PIP, 2nd to 5th MTPs, thumb IP, and wrists.
†Low positive: >ULN but <×3 ULN; high positive >×3 times ULN.

anti-CCP: anticitrullinated peptide antibody; CRP: C-reactive protein; ESR: erythrocyte sedimentation rate; IP: interphalangeal; MCP: metacarpal–phalangeal; MTP: metatarsal–phalangeal; PIP: proximal interphalangeal; RF: rheumatoid factor; ULN: upper limit normal.

INVESTIGATIONS
Laboratory
- General: Anemia and thrombocytosis (which parallel disease activity) are common. ESR and CRP are frequently elevated and may be helpful in tracking treatment response.
- Autoantibodies: anti-CCP and RF are both diagnostically and prognostically useful. Anti-CCP is approximately 98% specific and 70% sensitive. Despite its high specificity, anti-CCP is not useful as a general population screening test since the prevalence of RA is only 1%. The specificity of RF in RA is probably <50% unless used in select populations (patients with inflammatory arthritis), and has a sensitivity of ~80%. Finally, one-third of RA patients are positive for ANA and ANA has some correlation with severe disease.

Imaging
Plain radiography, particularly of the hands and feet, may be helpful diagnostically in evaluating for changes typical of RA and ruling out alternative diagnoses. Early X-ray changes include the development of periarticular osteopenia with the later development of marginal erosions. Radiographs of the C-spine are critical for the evaluation of possible cervical involvement including C1–C2 subluxation. Chest radiography and high-resolution computed tomography (CT) are helpful in evaluating for pulmonary involvement in RA. Routine dual-energy X-ray absorptiometry (DXA) is needed to assess bone mineral density status and fracture risk. The role of routine magnetic resonance imaging (MRI) and ultrasonography (US) in the detection of subclinical synovitis and bone erosions not visualized by plain radiography is currently being investigated.

HISTOLOGY
In RA, the primary site of inflammation is the synovium. Normal synovial lining is one to two cell layers thick; in RA it is often hypertrophied ~10-fold. Synovial lining hyperplasia, angiogenesis, and the infiltration of predominately CD4+ T cells, B cells, and macrophages (synoviocytes) are the hallmark.

PROGNOSIS
RA can be a devastating disease with increased morbidity as well as mortality. The primary cause of the excess mortality associated with RA is systemic inflammation and its devastating effects on the vascular endothelium (and increased cardiovascular disease). Factors associated with increased mortality in RA include advancing age, male gender, nodules, seropositivity, greater inflammation, lower functional scores, and prednisone use. Importantly, dramatic improvements in therapies and early diagnosis have occurred in the last 15 years; therefore, the prognosis for patients diagnosed early and managed appropriately by primary care doctors in collaboration with rheumatologists, is excellent.

MANAGEMENT
The keys to successful management of RA are shown in *Table 9*. It is critical to start disease-modifying antirheumatic drug (DMARD) therapy early, within the first few months of disease, and to escalate the dose, add other DMARDs when necessary, and treat to a target of low level of disease activity. There is currently some debate over what the target should be – a low level of disease activity or full remission. Obviously, remission is the ultimate goal if it is obtainable without significant drug-related toxicity or the risk of this toxicity. Disease activity level is determined by composite criteria that usually include tender and swollen joint counts, patient-reported global disease activity, and laboratory measures of inflammation such as ESR or CRP.

Table 9 Key points regarding the management of rheumatoid arthritis

Diagnose early and start disease-modifying, antirheumatic drug (DMARD) therapy
Treat to a target
Use combinations of DMARDs if needed
Aggressively treat co-morbid conditions

For initial therapy, multiple conventional and biologic DMARDs are available for use (*Table 10*). For most patients, methotrexate (MTX) is not only the initial treatment of choice but is the foundation for combination therapy when necessary. MTX has been shown to improve significantly both cardiovascular and overall survival. MTX is extremely well tolerated when used once weekly and given with folic acid. MTX dramatically improves clinical and radiographic outcomes in RA. Hydroxychloroquine (HCQ) and sulfasalazine (SSZ) are the next two most frequently used DMARDs and work particularly well in combination with MTX. If initial mono-DMARD therapy does not result in the patient achieving the target, combination therapy is used. MTX is usually continued and conventional or biologic drugs (*Table 10*) are added. Currently, attempts to combine biologic drugs have resulted in unacceptably high rates of toxicities, especially infections, and therefore, biologic combinations are contraindicated.

For established disease, when patients have active disease despite MTX, then either adding HCQ and SSZ or a TNF-inhibitor is the treatment of choice for most patients. It is worth noting that all of the TNF-inhibitors work best when used in combination with MTX. If patients fail a TNF-inhibitor, then abatacept, rituximab, or tocilizumab should be considered.

Table 10 Conventional and biologic disease-modifying antirheumatic drugs (DMARDs) used to treat rheumatoid arthritis

Conventional DMARDs	Biologic DMARDs
Methotrexate	Etanercept (TNF receptor)
Hydroxychloroquine	Infliximab (anti-TNF)
Sulfasalazine	Anakinra (IL- receptor antagonist)
Leflunomide	Adalimumab (anti-TNF)
Gold	Abatacept
Azathioprine	Rituximab (anti-CD20)
Cyclosporine	Certolizumab (anti-TNF)
Minocycline	Golimumab (anti-TNF)
Glucocorticoids	Tocilizumab (anti-IL-6 receptor)

IL: interleukin; TNF: tumor necrosis factor.

Gout

DEFINITION

Gout or gouty arthritis is an inflammatory arthritis resulting from hyperuricemia and the deposition of monosodium urate (MSU) crystals in the synovium and surrounding tissues.

EPIDEMIOLOGY AND ETIOLOGY

Gout affects up to 4% of the general population and represents the most common form of inflammatory arthritis affecting men over the age of 40 years. Gout risk increases with advancing age affecting more than 10% of men over the age of 65 years. Although approximately four to five times more common in men than women, gout incidence increases in women following menopause with women comprising one-quarter to one-third of gout cases in the elderly.

Chronic hyperuricemia (serum urate concentrations >6.8 mg/dl [0.4 mmol/l]) typically precedes gout by 20 to 30 years and is observed in ~20% of the population. Factors associated with hyperuricemia and gout are shown in *Table 11*.

PATHOGENESIS

Uric acid is the byproduct of purine metabolism with xanthine oxidase as the rate-limiting enzyme in this pathway. Hyperuricemia is due to an imbalance between urate synthesis and renal excretion with under-excretion characterizing a majority of cases (~80%). Uricase, absent in humans but present in other mammalian species, further metabolizes uric acid into highly soluble allantoin. Rarely, gout can be caused by known genetic mutations that lead to either underexcretion (e.g. familial juvenile hyperuricemic nephropathy) or overproduction (e.g. hypoxanthine phosphoro ribosyl transferase [HPRT] deficiency or Lesch–Nyhan disease). In a minority of hyperuricemic individuals, MSU crystals precipitate in joints or surrounding tissues leading to gouty inflammation. MSU is absent from normal joint fluid, and the inflammation invoked via MSU deposition is neutrophil-dependent. Gouty inflammation is characterized by the expression of several proinflammatory cytokines (IL-1, TNF-α, IL-6, and IL-8), and chemokines in addition to inflammasomes. MSU crystals have been shown *in vitro* to activate both the classic and alternative complement pathways.

Table 11 Factors associated with the risk of hyperuricemia and gout

Increased serum urate and increased gout risk
  Sociodemographics: Older age, male gender, select race/ethnicity (higher in African-Americans than Caucasians; high gout incidence among Pacific Islanders)
  Dietary and health behavior factors
    High purine meats and seafood
    Beer and liquor
  Co-morbidities
    Obesity
    Metabolic syndrome
    Hypertension
    Renal insufficiency
    Conditions characterized by increased cell turnover (lymphoproliferative malignancy, psoriasis)
  Medications
    Low-dose aspirin
    Diuretics (e.g. thiazides and loop diuretics)
    Calcineurin inhibitors (e.g. cyclosporine)
    Niacin
    Ethambutol and pyrazinamide

Decreased serum urate and decreased gout risk
  Dietary and health behavior factors
    Dairy products
    Vitamin C
    Coffee
  Medications
    High-dose aspirin
    Fenofibrate
    Losartan
    Estrogen replacement therapy

CLINICAL HISTORY

The natural course of gout includes four stages:

1 Asymptomatic hyperuricemia – starting in adolescence in men and postmenopausal in women and lasting 20–30 years; it is characterized by an absence of clinical manifestations.

2 Acute flares – resulting in acute joint inflammation caused by the deposition of MSU crystals; recognizing wide variability, gout onset is typically in the third to fourth decade in men and follows menopause in women.

3 Intercritical segments – the intervals between acute flares, which may initially last years, but when untreated often become shorter and shorter over time.

4 Advanced/tophaceous gout – typically occurs after years of uncontrolled gout/ hyperuricemia; characterized by the presence of tophaceous deposits (tophi) in the synovium and other tissues; it can closely mimic other forms of chronic inflammatory arthritis (e.g. RA).

PHYSICAL EXAMINATION

Physical findings in acute gout include evidence of arthritis (swelling, erythema, and tenderness) that may be 'intensely inflammatory'. Commonly affected joints/joint areas include the feet (MTP joints, midfoot), ankle, knee, wrist, elbow (including olecranon bursitis), and small joints of the hand. Acute arthritis is monoarticular in most cases (~80%), but can be polyarticular. First MTP involvement is the initial joint to be involved in ~50% of cases and occurs in ~90% of affected individuals sometime in the course of the disease. Acute gout can result in an overlying aseptic cellulitis in addition to low-grade fevers. Findings in chronic gout can include tophi and joint deformities resulting from suboptimal treatment and subsequent degenerative changes. Tophi are most commonly seen over the extensor surface of the elbow but can be observed in other locations (prepatellar bursa, outer ear, overlying small joints of the hand). Chronic deformities, including ulnar drift and palmar subluxation, along with the presence of subcutaneous nodules, can mimic RA (**42–45**).

DIFFERENTIAL DIAGNOSIS

In patients with a compatible clinical history, the differential diagnosis of acute gout includes arthritis due to infection (including gonococcal and nongonococcal arthritis), alternative crystalline athridites (most commonly pseudogout [calcium pyrophosphate dehydrate, CPPD], less commonly calcium hydroxyapatite deposition), and other rheumatic conditions that cause an inflammatory arthritis (RA, reactive arthritis [ReA], lupus, and so on). As noted above, chronic gout can closely mimic RA. Other rheumatic conditions that can result in arthritis and nodules include rheumatic fever, lupus, and multicentric reticulohistiocytosis.

INVESTIGATIONS

Aspiration

Synovial fluid analysis is the cornerstone of acute gout diagnosis (see Histology). Crystals can be aspirated from previously inflamed joints during an intercritical period if the patient has not been treated with urate-lowering therapy. While MSU crystals can be visualized using plain light microscopy, polarized microscopy is required for definitive identification. Aspirates from tophi can also be diagnostic. Biopsy/surgical specimens should be placed in alcohol preservative rather than formaldehyde since the latter will dissolve MSU in solution. Synovial fluid gram stain and culture are imperative to rule out infection, which can rarely occur simultaneously with acute gout.

Imaging

Imaging is not typically helpful in the diagnosis of acute gout but may be helpful in ruling out alternative diagnoses. In chronic gout, radiographs may reveal characteristic findings including bony erosions characterized by 'overhanging' edges and relatively well-preserved joint spaces (**46**).

Laboratory

A normal serum urate (<6.8 mg/dl [0.4 mmol/l]) does not rule out acute gout nor is hyperuricemia diagnostic of gout. Of marginal clinical utility, a 24-hour urine collection for total urate can help to differentiate underexcretors from overproducers of uric acid. Serum creatinine should be measured to assess for secondary gout related to renal insufficiency and to help guide choice/dose of urate-lowering therapy.

HISTOLOGY

Arthrocentesis and synovial fluid analysis in acute gout generally yield an inflammatory joint fluid (>2000–50 000 white blood cells [WBCs] per µl with predominance of neutrophils) with intra-and/or extracellular MSU crystals visualized under polarized microscopy. Intracelluar MSU crystals are pathognomonic of gout. MSU crystals have a needle-shaped morphology and are negatively birefringent, appearing yellow with a parallel orientation to light from the red compensator

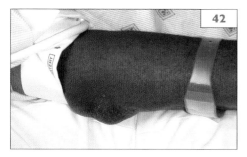

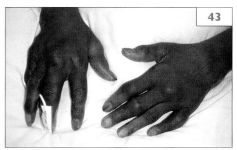

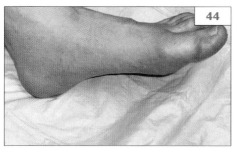

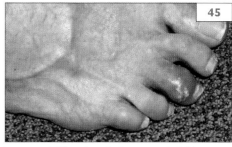

42–45 Clinical findings in gout: tophus over right olecranon (**42**); polyarticular gout mimicking rheumatoid arthritis (**43**); acute gout of the left first metatarsal–phalangeal joint, also known as podagra (**44**); acute gout with drainage of urate from third toe mimicking acute infectious process (**45**). (Courtesy of Dr GF Moore.)

46 Hand radiograph in patient with chronic tophaceous gout, showing characteristic gouty erosion of the distal first proximal phalanx (arrow).

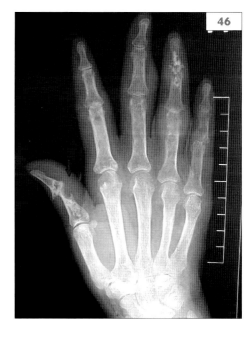

(**47**). In contrast, pseudogout/CPPD crystals are generally rhomboidal (although rarely rod-shaped) and weakly positively birefringent (blue when parallel to light from red compensator). Rarely, MSU form birefringent spherules.

PROGNOSIS

When managed optimally, gout has an excellent overall prognosis. Urate-lowering therapy and chronic maintenance of serum urate concentrations below 6.0 mg/dl (0.36 mmol/l) can eliminate gout flares over time. With suboptimal management, gout can lead to significant disability and work loss. While gout *per se* does not result in decreased survival, associated co-morbid conditions (metabolic syndrome and cardiovascular disease) must be aggressively addressed to minimize their impact on both morbidity and mortality.

MANAGEMENT

Major tenets include the treatment of acute gout flares and the use of urate-lowering medication to reduce gout flare frequency and to prevent joint damage.

Acute flares can be treated with NSAIDs, colchicine and/or glucocorticoids (GCs) (with adrenocorticotrophic hormone [ACTH] as an alternative); IV colchicine should be used only with great caution given its relatively narrow therapeutic window.

Urate-lowering drugs should be initiated in patients with: 1) tophi; 2) radiographic damage; or 3) frequent gout flares. Urate-lowering medications should not be started during acute flares, but once initiated, are generally required lifelong; the goal of therapy is to reduce and maintain serum urate levels below 6.0 mg/dl (0.36 mmol/l)); 'rebound flares' with rapid urate lowering can be minimized with anti-inflammatory prophylaxis (e.g. colchicine 0.6 mg qd to bid or naprosyn 375–500 mg bid), typically for a period of at least 3–6 months after starting a urate-lowering treatment. Approved urate-lowering drugs include uricosuric agents (probenecid), xanthine oxidase inhibitors (allopurinol and febuxostat), and pegloticase (see below).

Uricosurics are generally ineffective for patients with significant renal impairment (glomerular filtration rate [GFR] <50 ml/min). Although not universally available, both benzbromarone and sulfinpyrazone are uricosurics that have been used effectively as urate-lowering agents in the treatment

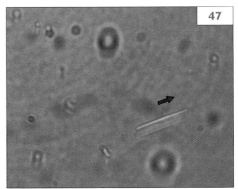

47 Polarized microscopy of gouty synovial fluid, showing characteristic intracellular negatively birefringent monosodium urate (MSU) crystals; MSU crystals are needle shaped and appear yellow when parallel to the light from the red compensator (arrow). (Courtesy of Dr GF Moore.)

of gout. In contrast to more widely available uricosurics, benzbromarone may be effective in the context of renal insufficiency although there have been rare cases of hepatotoxicity observed with its use.

Pegloticase (a pegylated recombinant uricase enzyme) is the latest form of drug to be released to lower urate in patients with otherwise treatment refractory gout (those intolerant to or unable to achieve treatment responses with more conventional therapies). Associated co-morbidities including hyperlipidemia, diabetes, hypertension, and cardiovascular disease should be aggressively evaluated and treated.

CPPD deposition, pseudogout, and chondrocalcinosis

DEFINITION
Calcium pyrophosphate dehydrate (CPPD) deposition encompasses several entities including 1) acute synovitis (pseudogout); 2) chronic pyrophosphate arthropathy; 3) acute pseudogout superimposed on chronic arthropathy; and 4) asymptomatic chondrocalcinosis. Pseudogout is an acute inflammatory arthritis related to formation and deposition of CPPD crystals in articular hyaline and fibrocartilage. Chronic pyrophosphate arthropathy refers to structural joint damage secondary to long-standing CPPD. Chondrocalcinosis is cartilagenous calcification due to CPPD evident pathologically and radiographically, which may be asymptomatic.

EPIDEMIOLOGY AND ETIOLOGY
The incidence and prevalence of symptomatic CPPD/pseudogout are not known. Most epidemiological surveys have examined the frequency of chondrocalcinosis, based on radiographic findings or postmortem examination (known to be much more common than pyrophosphate arthropathy or acute pseudogout). Reported prevalence varies widely based on the population and site (knee *vs.* other joints) examined. Chondrocalcinosis is more common with advanced age, with a prevalence ranging from 2% to 10% in patients below the age of 75 and as high as 30–60% above the age of 85 years. It is estimated that only ~25% of patients with CPPD deposits develop symptoms, the rest remain asymptomatic and evidence of disease found only on autopsy or radiographically. There also is an association of CPPD deposition with select metabolic diseases thought to be related to 'altered' calcium or inorganic pyrophosphate metabolism. Examples of such metabolic diseases that predispose to CPPD deposition include hyperparathyroidism, hypothyroidism, hypophosphatasia, hemochromatosis, and hypomagnesemia ('the Hs'). There is a genetic predisposition to develop pseudogout among certain ethnic groups. Early-onset chondrocalcinosis in select populations may be inherited as an autosomal dominant trait, linked to chromosomes 8q or 5p.

PATHOGENESIS
The mechanisms for pseudogout and chronic pyrophosphate arthropathy are thought to be different, although the pathogenesis of the latter is not well understood. Listed below are the ways in which acute pseudogout results in inflammation and articular damage.
- Activation of the direct complement system through immunoglobulin (Ig) G, and indirect complement system, producing complement breakdown products.
- Activation of Hageman factor which leads to production of mediators like bradykinin and kallikrein.
- Direct membrane activation of neutrophils leading to release of inflammatory mediators.
- Secretion of IL-1, TNF, IL-6.
- Mechanical effect with wear and tear at cartilage–cartilage interface with crystals present.
- Shedding of crystals into synovial fluid from deposits within cartilage causing further activation of neutrophils.

CLINICAL HISTORY AND PHYSICAL EXAMINATION
CPPD deposition is asymptomatic in a vast majority, resulting in chondrocalcinosis. It can however manifest symptomatically in two common ways:
- Pseudogout: Acute and intermittent attacks of arthritis; symptoms often peak within 6–24 hours of onset; usually self-limiting, and resolve within 1–2 weeks.
  - Intense articular inflammation (pain, swelling, erythema, tenderness).
  - Knee most commonly affected, followed by the wrist, shoulder, ankle, and elbow.
- Chronic pyrophosphate arthropathy (or pseudo-osteoarthritis); indolent course; signs and symptoms may suggest systemic inflammatory arthritis (reports of morning stiffness and pain); can be complicated by superimposed acute attacks.
  - Targets same joints as pseudogout; may also affect MCP joints in the hand; second/third MCP involvement is characteristic (but not diagnostic)

of overlapping hemochromatosis; history/examination may mimic OA; can also have pseudorheumatoid appearance with ulnar drift and MCP subluxation (**48**).

DIFFERENTIAL DIAGNOSIS

Approximately 5% of patients with CPPD deposition (particularly those with chronic arthropathy) may have symptoms that mimic RA, a presentation referred to as pseudo-RA. They may have morning stiffness, synovitis, and involvement of symmetric small joints, with elevated inflammatory indices. Gout and septic arthritis must always be considered in the differential diagnosis, particularly in the context of acute pseudogout. Deposition of the crystals in the ligamentum flavum can rarely cause symptoms that mimic meningitis. Involvement of the cervical spine with inflammatory changes at C1–C2 articulation has also been rarely reported. It is important to recognize the substantial overlap of CPPD deposition with OA in many patients. Clinical hints suggesting the presence of CPPD (rather than OA alone) include: involvement of uncommon joints for OA (e.g. MCPs or elbow), radiographic appearance (e.g. radiocarpal narrowing), prominent subchondral cysts, severely progressive degenerative findings, variable and inconsistent osteophyte formation, and tendon calcifications. Other calcium crystal deposition diseases can result in chronic arthropathy, most notably those involving calcium hydroxyapatite (where crystals are not readily seen under polarized microscopy). Calcium hydroxyapatite deposition is increased in the context of chronic kidney disease and can result in Milwaukee shoulder syndrome (chronic rotator cuff disease with advanced glenohumeral degenerative disease).

INVESTIGATIONS

Synovial fluid analysis from joint aspiration is the cornerstone of acute pseudogout diagnosis (see Histology) and is essential to rule out other causes of acute arthritis (e.g. septic arthritis or gout) (**49**).

Radiographic punctate and linear densities in fibrocartilaginous tissue or hyaline articular cartilage are diagnostic of chrondrocalcinosis while diffuse calcification of ligaments or bursa may also occur (**50**). These may be visible on plain radiograph and may also be demonstrated on CT, US, and MRI. Radiographic findings may also include secondary degenerative changes with

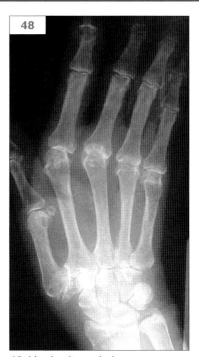

48 Hand radiograph showing degenerative changes, ulnar drift at the metacarpophalangeal joints in patient with pseudorheumatoid presentation of chronic pyrophosphate arthropathy with documented calcium pyrophosphate dehydrate on synovial fluid analysis.

notable involvement in joints that would be atypical for primary OA (**51**).

In patients with early onset arthritis (age <55 years), polyarticular arthritis, recurrent attacks, a workup to rule out metabolic diseases with calcium, magnesium, phosphorus levels, TSH, alkaline phosphatase, ferritin, transferrin saturation, and liver function tests should be considered. Diagnostic criteria are shown in *Table 12*.

HISTOLOGY

Synovial fluid analysis in CPPD deposition often reveals turbid fluid, which may also be blood stained, with decreased viscosity. Analysis of fluid typically shows an inflammatory WBC count

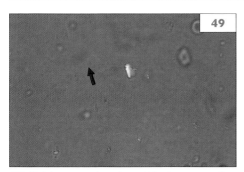

49 Calcium pyrophosphate dehydrate crystal visualized under polarized microscopy; note typical rhomboidal morphology and weak positive birefringence, appearing blue in parallel to the axis of the red compensator (arrow). (Courtesy of Dr GF Moore.)

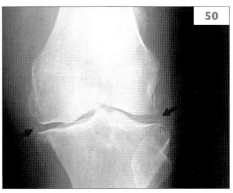

50 Chondrocalcinosis of the meniscal cartilage on knee radiograph (arrows), most notable in the lateral compartment.

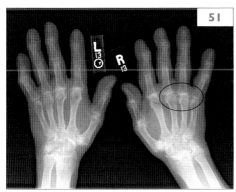

51 Radiograph of the hands and wrists from a patient with advanced calcium pyrophosphate dehydrate deposition resulting in chronic pyrophosphate arthropathy. Radiographs demonstrate marked diffuse secondary degenerative changes (with involvement of radiocarpal joints and metacarpal–phalangeal joints) and chondrocalcinosis of the triangular ligament in the left wrist (arrow). Note the presence of hooked osteophytes on the radial aspect of the MCP joints (circle). (Courtesy of Dr GF Moore.)

Table 12 Diagnostic criteria for calcium pyrophosphate dehydrate (CPPD)

Diagnostic criteria*
1. Demonstration of CPPD crystals in tissue or synovial fluid by definitive means, which include direct observation under microscope, X-ray defraction, or chemical analysis
2A. Identification of monoclinic or triclinic crystals showing no or weakly positive birefringence by compensated polarized light microscopy
2B. Presence of typical calcifications on X-ray (most commonly observed in the knee or triangular ligament in the wrist)
3A. Acute arthritis especially involving the knees and other large joints, with or without concomitant hyperuricemia
3B. Chronic arthritis involving the knee, hip, wrist, carpus, shoulder, elbow, or MCP joint ± acute exacerbations

*Patients should have the following for diagnosis:
Definitive disease: Criteria 1 or 2A + 2B must be fulfilled
Probable disease: Criteria 2A or 2B must be fulfilled
Possible disease: Criteria 3A or B or in any combination should alert the clinician to the possibility of underlying CPPD deposition

(ranging between >2000–50 000 cells per μl with a predominance of PMNs), but the WBC count can vary from inflammatory to noninflammatory cell counts. Polarized light microscopy demonstrates weakly positive birefringent rhomboid-shaped crystals (**49**).

PROGNOSIS

When managed optimally, CPPD deposition generally has an excellent overall prognosis. While CPPD deposition *per se* does not result in decreased survival, associated metabolic conditions (if present) need to be aggressively addressed to minimize their impact on both morbidity and mortality. While anti-inflammatory agents can be quite effective in the treatment of intermittent pseudogout attacks, the treatment of chronic pyrophosphate arthropathy has proven far more challenging. In some patients, progressive arthropathy can lead to rapidly progressive degenerative arthritis, leading to significant functional impairment.

MANAGEMENT

In acute pseudogout, anti-inflammatory agents including NSAIDs, systemic GCs, and colchicine may be effective, particularly when administered early in the course of an attack. Acetaminophen (paracetamol) and other analgesics may provide additional symptomatic relief. Optimal clinical improvement in pseudogout can be achieved by therapeutic aspiration of the joint with intra-articular steroid administration, an option that is particularly helpful with monoarticular flares. In patients with chronic pyrophosphate arthropathy, long-term management includes both aerobic and muscle strengthening exercises, maintenance of range of motion (ROM), weight loss in the obese, assistive devices, and less often surgical interventions such as synovectomy or arthroplasty. Any underlying metabolic condition should be treated aggressively, recognizing that the course of chronic arthropathy in the context of hemochromatosis is not altered even with optimal phlebotomy or iron chelation. DMARDs, including MTX and HCQ, have been used to treat chronic pyrophosphate arthropathy with anecdotal success.

Adult-onset Still's disease

DEFINITION

Adult-onset Still's disease (AOSD) is a rare systemic inflammatory disorder of unknown etiology characterized by daily high, spiking fevers, evanescent rash, and arthritis.

EPIDEMIOLOGY AND ETIOLOGY

AOSD is rare and there is no consensus on its incidence and prevalence. Several reviews suggest that women might be affected slightly more often than men, although men may be more likely to present at a younger age. The yearly incidence has been estimated to be 0.16 per 100 000 population. It usually occurs in younger people with a bimodal incidence peak at ages 15–25 and 36–46 years. Several cases have been reported after the age of 60 years.

The etiology of AOSD is not well understood, although 'physiological stressors' during the year preceding AOSD have been associated with disease.

PATHOGENESIS

It is believed currently that the immune response is dysregulated in AOSD patients. Although the exact mechanisms underpinning the occurrence of immune dysregulation are still unclear, a predominance of T-helper cytokines (Th1) have been reported in the blood and tissues of patients with active AOSD. IL-2, IL-6, IL-8, IL-18, and TNF-α all appear to be over-expressed in sera and effected tissues in AOSD. These proinflammatory cytokines in turn promote B cell IgG2a production, the activation of both macrophages and natural killer (NK) cells, and promote cell-mediated immunity.

CLINICAL HISTORY AND PHYSICAL EXAMINATION

AOSD typically manifests as a triad of symptoms that include high-spiking fevers, a characteristic rash, and arthritis/arthralgias.

Fever is quotidian (spiking, returning to normal, **52**) or double-quotidian (two fever spikes per day); generally ≥39°C, transient, lasting typically <4 hours. Temperature swings can be dramatic, with highest temperatures in the late afternoon or early evening. Temperatures normalize in 80% of patients untreated with antipyretics. It can also present as fever of unknown origin (FUO) and myalgias commonly accompany fever.

Rash appears as evanescent, salmon-pink color and macular or maculopapular eruptions (**53**); it commonly involves proximal limbs and trunk, less often the palms and soles. Rash is most prominent during fevers and can be mildly pruritic. Rash is frequently misdiagnosed as a drug reaction. Koebner phenomenon may be present (cutaneous eruptions elicited by stroking the skin).

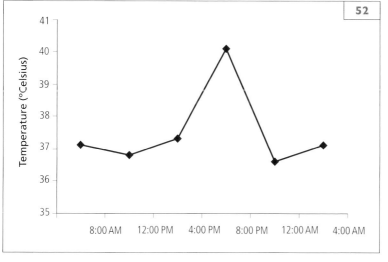

52 A quotidian fever pattern in a patient with adult-onset Still's disease; note marked temperature spike with a rapid return to normal.

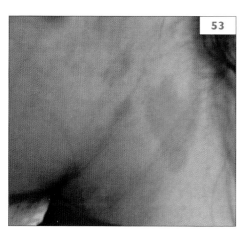

53 Evanescent, salmon-pink rash in a young woman with adult-onset Still's disease; rash may be macular or papular with areas of confluence and varies markedly in its distribution over the trunk and extremities and often accompanies episodes of fever. (Courtesy of Dr Adam Reinhardt.)

Arthralgias and arthritis are found in the majority of patients (64–100%). The most commonly affected joints include knees, wrists, ankles, and elbows, although involvement of the shoulders, PIPs, DIPs, MCPs, MTPs, temperomandibular (TMJ) joints, and hips have been described. Affected joints are usually symmetric, polyarticular, with increased arthralgias with fevers.

Other common clinical manifestations include sore throat, lymphadenopathy, hepatosplenomegaly, pleuritis, and pericarditis. AOSD affects numerous organs and the full constellation of clinical features may not be present at onset, but may evolve over weeks to months in an untreated patient.

DIFFERENTIAL DIAGNOSIS

The clinical presentation of AOSD is heterogeneous, and the spectrum of differential diagnoses to be considered is broad. AOSD is a diagnosis of exclusion and entities that must be considered in the differential diagnosis include:

- Infectious disorders (hepatitis B and C, rubella, parvovirus, coxsackie, Epstein–Barr virus, cytomegalovirus, human immunodeficiency virus (HIV), subacute endocarditis (SBE), chronic meningococcemia, tuberculosis, Lyme disease, syphilis, rheumatic fever, sepsis).
- Neoplastic disorders (leukemia, lymphoma, angioblastic lymphadenopathy).
- Autoimmune disorders (systemic lupus erythematosus [SLE], mixed connective tissue disease [MCTD], polymyositis, dermatomyositis), Behçet's disease, vasculitis).
- Granulomatous disorders (sarcoidosis, Crohn's disease, idiopathic granulomatous hepatitis).
- Autoinflammatory syndromes.
- Kikuchi's lymphadenitis.
- Sweet's syndrome.
- Macrophage activation syndrome.
- Schnitzler's syndrome.

Diagnostic criteria have been proposed by several authors; the Yamaguchi criteria are shown in *Table 13*. Most patients do not present with the full-blown syndrome. Even a typical patient may take weeks or months to satisfy the diagnostic criteria.

INVESTIGATIONS

Elevations in ESR and/or CRP are nearly universal. Leukocytosis, thrombocytosis, and low-grade anemia are common. Liver function tests may be elevated. RF and ANA tests are generally negative. A characteristic laboratory abnormality

Table 13 The Yamaguchi classification criteria for the diagnosis of adult-onset Still's disease (AOSD)*

Criteria
Major criteria

Fever >39°C, lasting >1 week

Arthralgias lasting >2 weeks

Typical rash

Leukocytosis >10 000/mm^3 (>80% granulocytes)

Minor criteria

Sore throat

Lymphadenopathy and/or splenomegaly

Liver dysfunction

Negative RF and negative ANA

Exclusions

Infections (especially sepsis and infectious mononucleosis)

Malignancy (especially lymphoma)

Alternative rheumatic diseases (e.g. polyarteritis nodosa and rheumatoid vasculitis with extra-articular features)

* Diagnosis of AOSD requires five or more criteria including two or more major criteria. In 2002, a new set of criteria were proposed by Faultrel, which contained two new laboratory markers: elevations in serum ferritin and a decreased glycosylated fraction of ferritin. Yamaguchi criteria have a sensitivity of 96.2% and a specificity of 92.1%. ANA: antinuclear antibody; RF: rheumatoid factor.

is a highly elevated ferritin. Ferritin levels in AOSD are usually higher than those found in patients with other autoimmune or inflammatory diseases. In most studies, a threshold for serum ferritin levels of 1000 ng/ml has been used to suggest AOSD with levels as high 4000–30 000 ng/ml reported. Serum ferritin level correlates with disease activity and often normalizes when the disease goes into remission. A more specific diagnostic marker than ferritin may be its glycosylated fraction. In healthy subjects, 50–80% of ferritin is glycosylated. In inflammatory states, saturation of glycosylation mechanisms results in a decreased glycosylated fraction (often <20% in AOSD). With refractory or suboptimally treated disease, radiographic damage can occur (**54**). Other laboratory (i.e. urinalysis, blood cultures, and so on) and imaging studies (i.e. chest X-ray) are necessary to exclude other considerations in the differential diagnosis (see above).

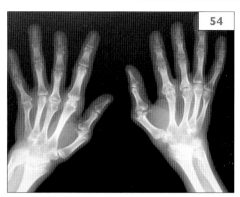

54 Progressive joint space narrowing in a pericapitate or carpometacarpal distribution, and ankylosis developing after 1.5–3 years found in subset of patients with adult onset Still's disease; note marked destructive changes in both wrists. (Courtesy of Dr GF Moore.)

HISTOLOGY
Although biopsies are not routine in AOSD, histology of involved skin shows perivascular inflammation of the superficial dermis with invasion of lymphocytes and histiocytes; immunofluorescence of the skin biopsy may show slight deposition of C3 and immunoglobulins. Analysis of synovial fluid shows marked elevation in leukocytes with a predominance of PMNs.

PROGNOSIS
The clinical course can often be categorized as one of three distinct patterns, each affecting about one-third of patients with AOSD.

The self-limited or monocyclic pattern is characterized by systemic symptoms (fever, rash, serositis, and organomegaly) occurring in a single episode. Most patients achieve remission within 1 year.

Patients with the intermittent or polycyclic systemic pattern experience recurrent flare, with or without articular symptoms. There is often complete remission between flares, which may be years apart and tend to be milder than the initial episode.

The chronic articular pattern is dominated by the articular manifestations that can be severe and lead to joint destruction. Patients with chronic articular disease generally have more disability and a worse prognosis.

MANAGEMENT
Treatment in AOSD is largely empirical, with data extrapolated from case reports, small case series, and retrospective studies. Corticosteroids are administered to a majority of patients at some point in the disease course, initial dose of 0.5–1.0 mg/kg/day prednisone equivalent. IV pulse methylprednisolone and dexamethasone have been used in refractory cases. DMARDs are often used in refractory disease or as 'steroid sparing' agents; MTX (weekly) is the most widely used DMARD. Biologic DMARDs (agents targeting TNF-α and IL-1) may be considered in refractory disease.

Septic arthritis

DEFINITION
Septic arthritis is an infection within a joint caused by the synovial seeding of micro-organisms, and is considered one of the most destructive forms of acute arthritis. Septic or infectious arthritis is commonly classified as typical bacterial arthritis (nongonococcal), gonococcal (GoC) or atypical septic arthritis.

EPIDEMIOLOGY
The rate of septic arthritis varies based on population demographics and underlying medical conditions. Elderly patients or those with RA, prosthetic joints, and severe medical co-morbidities are at much higher risk of septic (non-GoC) arthritis. Rates of septic arthritis in the general population range from two to five cases/100 000 person-years. However, in patients with RA or with prosthetic joints, that number increases to 28–70 cases/100 000 person-years. RA patients seem particularly affected due to factors including disease activity, underlying structural damage, and treatment modalities including corticosteroids, DMARDs, and biologic therapies. Septic arthritis most commonly affects the knees, but may affect any joint including the hips, ankles, wrists, shoulders, elbows, sternoclavicular, or sacroiliac joints.

GoC arthritis occurs in 1–3% of disseminated GoC (*Neisseria gonorrhea*) infections, with increased rates (2–4:1) noted in females. Females are more commonly afflicted due to asymptomatic gonorrheal infections and host changes related to menses.

PATHOGENESIS AND ETIOLOGY
Septic arthritis usually results from the hematogenous seeding of the synovium during episodes of bacteremia in a susceptible host. Less common causes of septic arthritis include local invasion via direct trauma, cellulitis, osteomyelitis, joint aspiration or injection, and joint replacement surgery. The incidence of septic arthritis after joint replacement or arthrocentesis is very small, occurring in less than 0.5% of patients. Most cases of non-GoC arthritis are due to staphylococci or streptococci, although many organisms have been implicated. *Staphylococcus aureus* is the most common and destructive organism causing non-GoC arthritis. *S. aureus* has acquired several virulence factors which account for its increased pathogenicity, including an enhanced ability to bind to local matrix proteins, activate local immune mediators, and avoid immune-mediated phagocytosis. Although reported, mycobacterial and fungal arthritis occur much less commonly than bacterial arthritis, most commonly in immunosuppressed individuals.

CLINICAL HISTORY
The clinical features of septic arthritis depend in part on the responsible organism and the individual patient. The classic presentation of non-GoC arthritis involves the abrupt onset on pain, swelling, and erythema in a single joint. These patients often appear ill, with fever and malaise common. Over 50% of all adult cases of non-GoC arthritis involve the knee, with hip involvement more common in children. Polyarticular involvement, while less common, is more likely to be seen in patients with underlying rheumatic diseases such as RA. Risk factors for the development of non-GoC arthritis include RA, intravenous drug abuse (particularly with involvement of the sacroiliac or sternoclavicular joints), immunosuppression, co-morbidities including malignancy, renal failure, and diabetes mellitus, and those patients with prosthetic joint replacement.

GoC arthritis is the most common acute arthritis seen in young, sexually active patients, with a higher incidence seen in young women. GoC arthritis classically presents with migratory arthritis or arthralgias, tenosynovitis, and rash. In these patients the tenosynovitis often affects multiple tendons, assisting with the diagnosis of GoC arthritis. Patients may have asymptomatic GoC infection, with arthritis or tenosynovitis as the first sign of dissemination. GoC arthritis may also present as an acute monoarthritis, usually involving the knee, without rash or tenosynovitis.

PHYSICAL EXAMINATION
Patients with acute bacterial arthritis often appear ill, and most will present with fever. Examination of the affected joint or joints often discloses a warm or hot, swollen, erythematous joint with a limited ROM. Patients may actively guard against movement of the affected joint. In patients with underlying rheumatic disease, it may be difficult to ascertain septic arthritis versus a flare of the underlying disease based on examination findings alone.

DIFFERENTIAL DIAGNOSIS

The differential diagnosis of an acute monoarthritis is broad, but initially should include trauma, infection, and crystal-induced arthritis (*Table 14*). The diagnosis of septic arthritis is dependent on aspiration and culture of synovial fluid from the affected joint or joints. In rare cases of fungal or mycobacterial arthritis, synovial biopsy may be necessary as synovial fluid cultures lack sensitivity for these organisms.

INVESTIGATIONS

It is imperative that all episodes of acute monoarthritis are investigated with arthrocentesis and synovial fluid analysis due to the high level of morbidity and mortality associated with septic arthritis (**55**). Synovial fluid analysis should include cell count with differential, Gram stain and culture, and crystal evaluation. Testing for protein, glucose, and lactate dehydrogenase is generally not recommended due to their poor sensitivity and specificity. Leukocyte counts in septic arthritis are generally elevated with counts often >50 000 WBC/mm^3 with a predominance of neutrophils. WBC counts may be much lower in cases of septic bursitis (**56**).

Blood cultures should be obtained in all patients with septic arthritis, and when GoC arthritis is suspected, cultures of the oropharynx, rectum, and genitourinary tract should be obtained. The yield of skin or tendon biopsies in patients with disseminated GoC is low, and is generally not recommended.

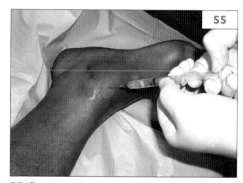

55 Patient with septic arthritis of the ankle; arthrocentesis revealed a grossly cloudy aspirate with subsequent cultures positive for *S. aureus*. (Courtesy of Dr GF Moore.)

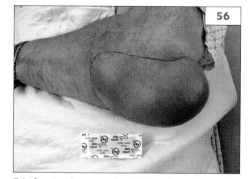

56 Septic olecranon bursitis; aspirate showed 17 000 leukocytes (98% polymorphonuclear cells) and culture was positive for *S. aureus*. (Courtesy of Dr Adam Burdorf.)

Table 14 Differential diagnosis of septic arthritis

Trauma

Gout

Pseudogout (CPPD)

Rheumatoid arthritis

Juvenile idiopathic arthritis

Seronegative spondyloarthropathy

Hemarthrosis

Radiographic evaluation of septic arthritis is recommended to rule out alternative diagnosis and provide for baseline evaluation in difficult to treat cases. In early disease, plain radiographs often show nonspecific evidence of inflammation including joint effusions and soft tissue swelling. Later in the course of the disease, destruction of both cartilage (manifesting as joint space narrowing) and bone may be seen (**57**).

HISTOLOGY

Synovial fluid in bacterial arthritis shows marked infiltration of WBCs with predominance of PMNs. With atypical infections (fungal or mycobacterial organisms) lymphocytes may predominate. As in other inflammatory arthritides, the involved synovium proliferates with time with marked infiltration of inflammatory cells.

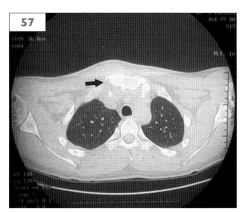

57 CT showing marked destructive bony changes secondary to septic arthritis of the sternoclavicular joint (arrow); the patient had a history of intravenous drug abuse.

PROGNOSIS

The prognosis of septic arthritis is dependent upon early evaluation and treatment. Patient factors, including co-morbid RA, immunosuppression, and co-morbid conditions all contribute to morbidity and mortality in septic arthritis. Polyarticular joint involvement has also been associated with greater overall mortality. In addition, pathogen virulence and the increasing emergence of antibiotic resistance will likely contribute to increased morbidity and mortality in the future.

MANAGEMENT

The management of septic arthritis is based on early antibiotic therapy and drainage of the affected joint. Early therapy is critical for preservation of the joint and reduction of the spread of infection.

Early joint aspiration may include arthrocentesis or surgical drainage and should be followed with repeat arthrocentesis to ensure resolution of the inflammatory process. The choice of drainage is controversial, with factors including access to orthopedic surgery, joint location, and patient co-morbid conditions factoring into the decision. Regardless of the decision, prompt drainage of the infected joints is mandatory. In patients with prosthetic joint infection, early orthopedic surgery involvement is necessary.

The choice of antibiotics is based on patient characteristics, clinical presentation, and Gram stain results with broad spectrum coverage favored initially. Initial empiric therapy with vancomycin and a third generation cephalosporin is generally adequate, with modification based on culture results. The duration of antibiotic coverage is unknown, but most experts recommend at least 14 days of IV therapy followed with 2–4 weeks of oral therapy based on sensitivity of the offending organism. In general, GoC arthritis responds to antibiotics quickly, with *S. aureus* arthritis exhibiting slower resolution and higher rates of relapse. Patients with GoC arthritis should be treated for possible concomitant chlamydial infection.

Viral arthritis

DEFINITION
Viral infections are commonly associated with self-limiting rheumatic complaints.While many viruses cause arthralgias or arthritis, this section highlights a few commonly implicated infections including parvovirus B19, rubella, hepatitis B, and hepatitis C.

Parvovirus B19

EPIDEMIOLOGY, ETIOLOGY, AND PATHOGENESIS
Parvovirus B19 is the most commonly seen viral arthritis, occurring frequently in schoolchildren and those with close contact with children. Most infections are characterized by seasonal variation (e.g. highest prevalence in winter and spring in North America and Europe), and are spread through respiratory secretions. It is estimated that most parvovirus B19 infections are asymptomatic and do not cause arthritis, especially in pediatric populations. As many as 70% of adult patients worldwide have serologic evidence of past parvovirus infection.

Parvovirus B19 is a small, nonenveloped, single-stranded deoxyribonucleic acid (DNA) virus of the family Parvoviridae, genus Erythrovirus. Parvovirus B19 consists of two structural proteins, VP1 and VP2, and a nonstructural protein NS1. Parvovirus replicates in erythroid precursors, and is often found in the bone marrow of infected patients. The signs and symptoms of rash and arthritis occur in the presence of antiparvovirus B19 IgM (at which time patients are no longer contagious). A small subset of patients develops chronic arthropathy, likely due to inappropriate production of antiparvovirus B19 IgG antibodies to VP1.

CLINICAL HISTORY AND PHYSICAL EXAMINATION
The clinical signs and symptoms of parvovirus B19 are varied and depend upon the age and immune status of the infected individual. B19 infection usually causes relatively benign flu-like symptoms, rash, and arthritis in immunocompetent hosts. Patients with underlying immunodeficiencies are more likely to suffer chronic infection-related illness, including pure red cell aplasia and pancytopenia. In children, B19 infection may result in Fifth's disease with a characteristic 'slapped cheek' appearance (**58**) while arthritis and generalized rash are more common in adults.

The incubation period of B19 infection is up to 2 weeks, and most symptomatic patients will exhibit nonspecific flu-like symptoms prior to the characteristic rash and arthritis. The arthritis of B19 is commonly seen in female patients and may mimic early, nonerosive RA. It typically presents as a symmetric arthritis involving the small joints of the hands, wrists, knees, ankles, and feet (**59**). Morning stiffness is common during this acute phase, and affected joints show typical inflammatory changes upon examination including warmth, erythema, and swelling. In most patients, the arthritis of B19 infection is self-limited.

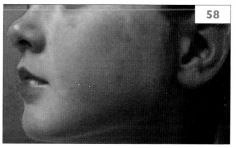

58 A young girl with parvovirus B19 infection and the characteristic 'slapped cheek' appearance.

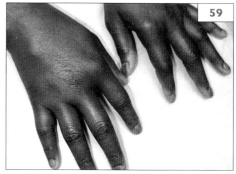

59 Inflammatory arthritis of the metacarpal–phalangeal and proximal interphalangeal joints bilaterally in a patient with parvovirus B19 infection. (Courtesy of Dr GF Moore.)

DIFFERENTIAL DIAGNOSIS

The differential diagnosis of acute arthritis with or without rash includes other viral infections, RA, and SLE.

INVESTIGATIONS

The onset of arthritis and rash correlates with the presence of IgM antibodies in the serum, assisting in the diagnosis of acute parvovirus infection. IgM antibodies are typically present for 2–6 months, and the presence of IgG antibodies without measureable IgM titers is indicative of previous infection. The presence of autoantibody, such as RF, anti-CCP antibody, or ANA may be indicative of alternative autoimmune etiologies.

PROGNOSIS AND MANAGEMENT

The prognosis of B19 infection depends on the age and immune status of the affected individual. Patients with underlying immunodeficiencies are at much higher risk of morbidity including hematologic effects and chronic, intermittent arthritis. The majority of patients will have a favorable prognosis without long-term complications.

The management of acute B19 arthritis involves symptomatic relief with NSAIDs and rest. In patients with chronic or life-threatening hematologic affects, the use of intravenous immunoglobulin (IVIG) is recommended.

Rubella

EPIDEMIOLOGY

Rubella virus was once a commonly seen infection; however, mass vaccination efforts have diminished its incidence in developed countries. Rubella is spread via respiratory secretions and is most commonly encountered in late winter and spring. Most infections involving arthritic complaints involve adult female patients and are self-limited in nature.

PATHOGENESIS AND ETIOLOGY

Rubella virus is a member of the togavirus family, genus Rubivirus, and is an enveloped, single-stranded ribonucleic acid (RNA) virus. Rubella initially infects nasopharyngeal cells, with evidence of spread to lymph nodes, synovial fluid, urine, and cerebrospinal fluid. Similar to other viral infections, the onset of arthritis corresponds to the production of antibodies, suggesting an immune complex process in the pathogenesis of disease.

CLINICAL HISTORY AND PHYSICAL EXAMINATION

Most infections with rubella virus are characterized by nonspecific, flu-like symptoms and rash. Arthralgias and arthritis are most commonly seen in adult women and often correspond with the onset of rash. Joint symptoms are typically short lived with most patients achieving resolution within days to weeks. Joints of the hands, wrists, knees, and ankles are often involved in a migratory pattern. These symptoms may be seen with both natural rubella infection and occurring weeks after vaccination.

DIFFERENTIAL DIAGNOSIS

The differential diagnosis of rubella arthritis includes RA, SLE, and other viral infections.

INVESTIGATIONS

The diagnosis of acute rubella arthritis involves the presence of antirubella IgM antibodies. As with other viral infections, the presence of IgG antibodies confers previous infection or vaccination. The culture of rubella from body fluid is not currently recommended due to poor sensitivity.

PROGNOSIS AND MANAGEMENT

The long-term prognosis of rubella arthritis is excellent. Most patients develop only mild self-limiting disease with only a small percentage developing chronic symptoms. The management of rubella arthritis consists of supportive care and the use of NSAIDs. Vaccination continues to be the best deterrent in the development of rubella infection and arthritis.

Hepatitis B and C

EPIDEMIOLOGY, ETIOLOGY AND PATHOGENESIS

Hepatitis B is a common infection seen worldwide, with the highest prevalence seen in developing countries. Vaccination and blood donation screening measures have reduced the incidence of acute hepatitis B infection in the US and Europe. In the US, hepatitis B is most commonly acquired through risky sexual behavior and intravenous drug abuse, while perinatal transmission remains a significant problem in many countries of Asia and Africa. The incidence of acute hepatitis B infection is less than 2 per 100 000 persons in the US.

Similar to hepatitis B infection, hepatitis C is a commonly encountered infection worldwide. Most cases are acquired by parenteral transmission with sexual transmission less commonly seen. In the US, the incidence of acute hepatitis C has fallen over the last 30 years due to better screening of blood products and educational programs aimed at reducing the spread of HIV and hepatitis C virus (HCV). The incidence of acute HCV infection is currently less than 0.5 cases per 100 000 persons, and most cases are related to intravenous drug abuse.

The pathogenesis of hepatitis B virus (HBV) and HCV-induced arthritis is related to immune complex deposition, the latter frequently in the context of cryoglobulin formation. Early viremia leads to the production of antihepatitis B surface antigen (HBsAg) antibodies and anti-HCV antibody with deposition into the synovium.

CLINICAL HISTORY AND PHYSICAL EXAMINATION

The rheumatic features of hepatitis B are usually confined to early HBV infection. Patients may notice the sudden onset of severe joint pain and swelling, most often affecting the hands and knees. While other joints may be involved, all rheumatic symptoms typically resolve prior to the onset of jaundice. Arthritis and arthralgias may persist in a minority of patients with chronic HBV infection. In addition to arthritis, HBV is associated with polyarteritis nodosa (PAN).

HCV is responsible for many rheumatic complaints including acute arthritis, arthralgias, myalgias, and the development of cryoglobulinemia. The arthritis of acute HCV infection may mimic that seen in acute HBV infection, but more commonly presents as arthralgias and myalgias. The development of chronic HCV infection is associated with both type II and type III cryoglobulinemia. Cryoglobulins are immunoglobulins which precipitate from serum when exposed to cold, and hepatitis C may be isolated from cryoprecipitate. Cryoglobulinemia is typically associated with skin, joint, renal, and neurologic symptoms and requires treatment of the underlying HCV infection. The arthritis is typically symmetric and nondeforming involving the hands, wrists, and knees.

DIFFERENTIAL DIAGNOSIS

The differential diagnosis of hepatitis B- or C-induced arthritis includes other infectious causes, SLE, and early RA.

INVESTIGATIONS

The diagnosis of acute HBV arthritis is made by detection of HBsAg in the serum. HCV infection is demonstrated through the detection of HCV viral load or the presence of anti-HCV antibodies in the serum. Patients with cryoglobulemia should undergo extensive evaluation for the presence of HCV, including evaluation of cryoprecipitate if needed. RF, particularly in low titer concentrations, may be positive in the context of HCV although anti-CCP antibodies are rarely seen as this autoantibody is nearly exclusive to RA.

PROGNOSIS AND MANAGEMENT

The management of acute HBV-related arthritis consists of conservative therapy and rest. The prognosis is good, with few patients experiencing long-term or recurrent arthritis.

Acute HCV arthritis is self-limiting and requires only conservative therapy. Patients with HCV-related cryoglobulinemia should consider treatment with appropriate antiviral therapy to decrease or eliminate the triggering antigen. In patients who fail antiviral therapy, the addition of immunosuppressive agents including corticosteroids, rituximab, or cyclophosphamide (CTX) may be beneficial. Chronic arthralgias complicating HCV are typically treated with a conservative approach.

Lyme disease

DEFINITION

Lyme disease is a tick-borne illness causing rash, flu-like symptoms, arthritis, and cardiac and neurologic symptoms (*Table 15*). It is caused by members of the spirochete species *Borrelia*, and spread by the bite of infected *Ixodes* ticks. In the US, most cases are confined to endemic areas.

EPIDEMIOLOGY AND ETIOLOGY

Lyme disease is a common tick-borne illness spread through the bite of the infected *Ixodes* ticks. First described in Lyme, Connecticut, US after an outbreak of arthritis in children, it is now commonly seen in the northeastern US (**60**), Europe, and Asia. In the US, it constitutes the most common tick-borne illness, with nearly 29 000 confirmed cases reported to the US Centers for Disease Control and Prevention in 2008. The genus *Borrelia burgdorferi sensu lato* contains three closely related members responsible for all cases of Lyme disease worldwide. In the US,

all cases of Lyme disease are caused by *B. burgdorferi sensu stricto*, acquired through the bite of infected *Ixodes scapularis* or *I. pacificus* ticks.

PATHOGENESIS

Small mammals constitute the main reservoir for *B. burgdorferi*, with the *Ixodes* tick species acting as the vector for human transmission. *Ixodes* ticks undergo three stages of maturation in their 2-year life cycle: larva, nymph, and adult. Larva may acquire the spirochete while feeding on infected small mammals. The larva molt into nymphs and remain inactive until the following spring (in North America and Europe), at which time they emerge to feed again. It is at this stage that human infections are most likely, as the nymphs actively feed at this time in preparation for the adult life stage (**61**). After reaching the adult cycle, ticks feed predominately on deer, which are not infected by *B. burgdorferi*. Deer do serve to promote the life cycle of the *Ixodes* tick species, but are not directly involved in the transmission of Lyme disease.

Table 15 Symptoms and stages of Lyme disease

Signs and symptoms	Early localized	Early disseminated	Late
Constitutional	Fever Malaise	Intense malaise and fatigue	
Skin	Erythema migrans (usually single lesion)	Multiple erythema migrans lesions	Acrodermatitis chronic atrophicans (Europe)
Cardiac		Atrioventricular nodal block Myocarditis	
Neurologic		Meningitis Headache Facial nerve palsy Radiculopathy Peripheral neuropathy Encephalopathy	Peripheral neuropathy Encephalopathy
Musculoskeletal	Polyarthralgias and myalgias	Migratory arthralgias or myalgias	Acute mono- or oligoarticular arthritis (≤10%) Chronic arthritis (rare)

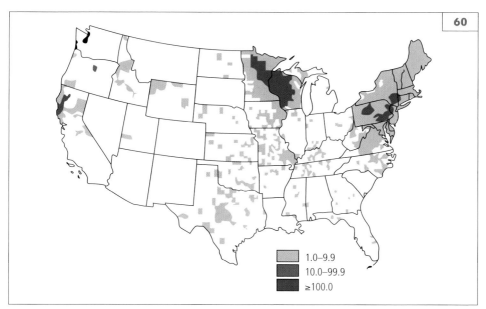

60

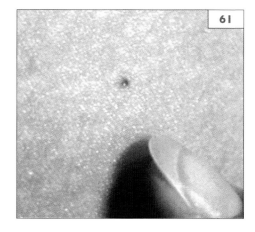

61

60 Average rate* of Lyme disease by county of residence† US 1992–2006‡ (Centers of Disease Control). *per 100 000 population; † county of residence available for 98.1% of cases reported during 1992–2006; ‡ during 2003, Pennsylvania reported 4722 confirmed cases and 1008 suspected cases.

61 Nymph stage of the *Ixodes scapularis* tick. (Copyright 2009 American College of Rheumatology. Used with permission.)

After the transmission of *Borrelia* sp. to the tick, the spirochete migrates to the salivary glands in preparation for entry into the human host. Spirochetes then multiply within the human skin prior to dissemination to other organs and tissues. The symptoms of Lyme disease are due to host inflammatory responses to the spirochete, rather than direct tissue damage.

CLINICAL HISTORY AND PHYSICAL EXAMINATION

Lyme disease, if left untreated, may progress through three stages: early localized disease, early disseminated disease, and late disease.

Early localized disease is characterized by the classic rash erythema migrans (EM) (**62**), which occurs in approximately 80% of infected individuals. EM is described as a rapidly expanding erythematous macule at the site of the tick bite, occurring within 3–30 days of the tick feeding. EM is classically referred to as a 'bull's eye' rash, due to the central clearing that may be seen in large lesions. EM is usually painless and should not be confused with a local tick bite reaction, which occurs earlier (within hours) and is often associated with pruritis and/or pain.

Early localized disease is commonly associated with flu-like symptoms, including fever, headache, myalgias, arthralgias, and malaise. It is noteworthy that early Lyme infections do not present with upper respiratory or gastrointestinal manifestations, helping to differentiate Lyme disease from other common viral ailments.

If early localized disease is left untreated, symptoms of early disseminated infection may begin within weeks. Symptoms may include intense fatigue with approximately 50% of patients developing multiple EM lesions. These secondary EM lesions are often found on the trunk, and are typically smaller than primary EM lesions. Patients with disseminated disease may exhibit cardiac manifestations, including atrioventricular conduction block and myocarditis. Disseminated disease may also affect both the peripheral and central nervous systems. Lyme disease is a common cause of unilateral or bilateral facial nerve palsy, although other cranial nerves may be affected. Less common manifestations of nervous system involvement include meningitis, radiculopathy, peripheral neuropathy, mononeuritis multiplex, and enchephalomyelitis.

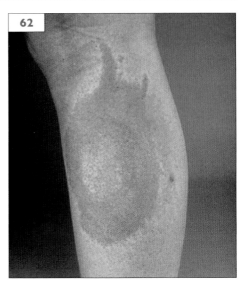

62 Classic erythema chronicum migrans lesion in Lyme disease.

Late disease is a rare manifestation, and occurs months to years after initial infection. It may present with rheumatic, neurologic, or skin disease. The classic skin finding in this stage is acrodermatitis chronic atrophicans, and is more commonly seen in European Lyme disease.

Patients with Lyme disease may complain of arthralgias or myalgias at any stage of disease, but true arthritis is considered a late complication. The arthritis of Lyme disease is seen in less than 10% of patients, and typically manifests as a mono- or oligoarthritis affecting large joints. Most cases involve the knee, although shoulder, elbow, wrist, hip, and TMJ joint involvement is also seen. Patients often present with a single warm, erythematous, and swollen joint. Interestingly, these effusions are typically less painful than other forms of infectious or inflammatory arthritis. If left untreated, effusions may last weeks to months with most patients experiencing fewer episodes over months to years.

A small minority of patients may develop 'post-Lyme' symptoms consisting of malaise, fatigue, myalgias, or short-term memory disturbances. These are typically short lived and do not require additional therapy. The term 'chronic Lyme disease' is usually avoided due to the lack of objective evidence for chronic infection in patients who have received standard antibiotic therapy.

DIFFERENTIAL DIAGNOSIS
The arthritis of Lyme disease must be differentiated from other causes of monoarticular arthritis including infection, trauma, and crystalline arthropathies (gout, CPPD). In addition, clinicians should consider seronegative spondylo-arthropathies, oligoarticular juvenile arthritis, and fibromyalgia in the differential of Lyme arthritis.

INVESTIGATIONS
In the presence of a classic EM lesion and an appropriate tick exposure history, further investigation is not needed in the diagnosis of Lyme disease. However, serologic evidence of disease is often necessary for accurate diagnosis when patients present without evidence of classic EM lesions. The serologic diagnosis is made utilizing a two-tiered approach with enzyme-linked immunosorbent assay (ELISA) and Western blot confirmation. The ELISA test has a high false-positive rate because it is derived from the whole antigen, and may have cross-reactivity with antibodies from other disease states, such as other borrelial and spirochetal infections or inflammatory diseases. The Western blot is more specific for *B. burgdorferi* antigens. Both tests must be positive for a diagnosis to be made. Positivity may persist for years after successful treatment. In addition, patients often exhibit nonspecific laboratory evidence of infection including elevated inflammatory markers and WBC counts.

Culture of *B. burgdorferi* from blood or other samples lacks sensitivity and is generally not recommended in the diagnosis of Lyme disease. It is possible to culture *B. burgdorferi* from the leading edge of EM lesions, although this is rarely needed in clinical practice.

Synovial fluid analysis will reveal marked inflammatory effusion, with an elevated WBC count similar to other etiologies of septic arthritis. Polymerase chain reaction (PCR) analysis of synovial fluid has high sensitivity in the detection of *B. burgdorferi* DNA and may be beneficial in the evaluation of Lyme arthritis.

MANAGEMENT AND PROGNOSIS
The management strategies for Lyme disease depend on the stage and symptoms targeted. Most patients can be managed with oral therapy, including patients with skin rash, arthritis, cardiac disease, or isolated cranial nerve palsies.

The management of early disease or EM is accomplished with oral doxycycline, amoxicillin, or cefuroxime. Patients with neurologic manifestations require up to 28 days of IV therapy with penicillin G or a third generation cephalosporin. The treatment of Lyme arthritis requires 28-day therapy with oral doxycycline, amoxicillin, or cefuroxime. In patients with recurrent arthritis or failure after oral therapy, an additional 14–28 days of oral or IV therapy is warranted.

In patients with ongoing arthritis despite two courses of antibiotics, further antibiotics therapy adds little benefit. The addition of NSAIDs , HCQ, or MTX may be of benefit in some patients. Some patients may require synovectomy for relief, but most cases of refractory arthritis improve with time. The prognosis of Lyme disease is generally favorable. Most patients with Lyme disease become asymptomatic with antibiotic therapy, and less than 10% of patients with Lyme arthritis develop refractory arthritis.

Rheumatic fever

DEFINITION

Acute rheumatic fever (ARF) is a multisystem inflammatory disease following pharyngeal infection with group A streptococcus.

EPIDEMIOLOGY

ARF is a common sequela of group A streptococcal infections in developing countries. It is estimated that the incidence of ARF approaches 20 cases/100 000 persons worldwide, with far lower rates seen in the US. Deaths related to ARF and rheumatic heart disease approach 250 000 worldwide each year. School-aged children are most affected, with socioeconomic and host factors contributing to its increased prevalence in the developing world.

PATHOGENESIS AND ETIOLOGY

ARF is an immune-mediated condition seen 2–3 weeks following pharyngeal group A streptococcal infection. The precise mechanism of disease is unknown, but thought to be related to host response to streptococcal pharyngitis. Genetic factors likely increase susceptibility, as evidenced by the high prevalence seen in certain populations. The role of group A streptococcus is based in part on epidemiologic evidence of ARF following epidemics of streptococcal pharyngitis, and the reduced incidence seen following treatment of documented streptococcal pharyngeal infections.

CLINICAL HISTORY AND PHYSICAL EXAMINATION

Arthritis is common occurring in ~75%, classically described as migratory and affecting the knees, ankles, wrists, and elbows. Erythema, warmth, and swelling of involved joints lasts days to approximately 1 week before moving to another region; left untreated, most cases spontaneously resolve in less than 4 weeks.

Carditis (~50%) represents the most severe complication; symptoms ranging from mild chest pain to severe valvulitis with congestive heart failure. All areas of the heart can be affected producing symptoms related to pericarditis, myocarditis, and endocarditis. Examination may reveal tachycardia, a new or changing murmur, friction rub, or signs of congestive heart failure.

Erythema marginatum is an uncommon manifestation of rheumatic fever often occurring early in the course of the disease, characteristically described as a pink, macular rash with central clearing involving the trunk and extremities, while sparing the face. It is often transient and may be exacerbated by heat or warm showers (**63**).

Syndenham chorea (St. Vitus dance) is a late manifestation occurring several months after initial infection. Symptoms include nonpurposeful, nonrhythmic movements with emotional distress. It generally requires no therapy and symptoms improve slowly over several months.

Subcutaneous nodules represent the least common major manifestation occurring in less than 1% of cases and require no specific treatment, resolving over time. There are correlations with severe carditis.

DIFFERENTIAL DIAGNOSIS

The differential diagnosis for patients without classic ARF is long and includes numerous conditions capable of inciting polyarthritis. In children, juvenile idiopathic arthritis (JIA), SLE, and poststreptococcal ReA should be considered. Patients with poststreptococcal ReA typically present earlier (within 2 weeks of infection) with severe arthritis which is relatively unresponsive to standard therapy used to treat ARF. In addition, poststreptococcal ReA generally lacks evidence of carditis.

INVESTIGATIONS

The diagnosis of ARF is generally made from a thorough history and physical examination and is based on the Jones Criteria which was most recently updated in 1992 (*Table 16*). There are no definitive diagnostic tests available to establish the diagnosis of ARF, but laboratory testing is helpful to demonstrate previous streptococcal infection. Numerous streptococcal antibodies are available including ASO, anti-DNAse B, and antistreptokinase, with peak titers seen in approximately 1 month. Most patients with ARF will also demonstrate nonspecific markers of inflammation, including an elevated ESR and CRP. All patients should undergo electro-cardiogram and chest radiograph evaluation to detect conduction defects or cardiomegaly due to asymptomatic carditis. Echocardiography increases the sensitivity of diagnosing carditis, and is a useful tool in the chronic management of patients with residual cardiac involvement.

HISTOLOGY

Histologically, the changes seen in ARF include edema, the infiltration of T cells and mononuclear cells, and localized necrosis. The presence of Aschoff bodies in myocardial tissue is indicative of ARF and is characterized by an area of central necrosis with surrounding histiocytes (Anitschkow cells) and lymphocytes (**64**).

63 Erythema marginatum is a rare manifestation of rheumatic fever characterized by a pink, irregular, centrifugally spreading rash with central clearing. It is typically seen on the trunk and upper extremities. (Copyright 2009 American College of Rheumatology. Used with permission.)

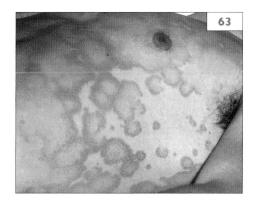

Table 16 Jones criteria used for the diagnosis of acute rheumatic fever*

Major criteria	Minor criteria
Carditis	Fever
Polyarthritis	Arthralgias
Chorea	Elevated acute phase reactants
Erythema marginatum	Prolonged PR interval on electrocardiogram
Subcutaneous nodules	

* Acute rheumatic fever is highly probable with evidence of preceding streptococcal infection and either two major OR one major and two minor criteria

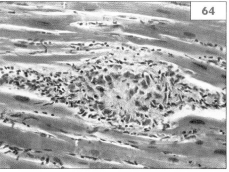

64 The Aschoff body, an area of central necrosis surrounded by histiocytes (Anitschkow cells) and lymphocytes, as seen in the myocardium of a patient with acute rheumatic fever. (Copyright 2009 American College of Rheumatology. Used with permission.)

MANAGEMENT AND PROGNOSIS

The management of ARF involves initial antibiotic therapy, anti-inflammatory agents, and prevention of future group A streptococcal infection.

All patients should receive initial treatment with penicillin (or erythromycin if penicillin allergic) at the time of diagnosis to eradicate group A streptococcal carriage. Penicillin may be administered as a single dose of intramuscular benzathine penicillin G, or as a 10-day course of oral penicillin V.

Anti-inflammatory agents are the primary therapeutic agents used in the treatment of ARF. Historically, aspirin (80–100 mg/kg/day in children, 4–8 g/day in adults) has been beneficial in the treatment of related arthritis or arthralgias. NSAIDs and corticosteroids are effective alternative agents, with corticosteroids often used in the management of patients with severe cardiac involvement. Anti-inflammatory agents often provide rapid symptomatic relief and normalization of acute-phase reactants.

Prevention of future group A streptococcal infections is imperative to prevent further cardiac complications. The American Heart Association has published recommendations regarding the appropriate use and duration of antibiotics for the secondary prevention of rheumatic fever. In patients with carditis and residual heart disease, prophylaxis should continue at least 10 years past the last episode, and until at least age 40 years.

Many experts recommend lifelong therapy in such patients. In those with a history of carditis without residual heart disease, prophylaxis should occur for 10 years or until age 21 years (whichever is longer). In patients without carditis, prophylaxis should occur for 5 years or until age 21 years (whichever is longer). Prophylaxis may be accomplished with either oral penicillin V twice daily or intramuscular injection of benzathine penicillin G at 3 or 4 week intervals.

The long-term prognosis of ARF is dependent upon the degree of cardiac involvement and the prevention of further episodes. To date, no medication or intervention during the acute episode has been shown to definitively prevent long-term cardiac complications; however, prevention of future episodes of ARF is paramount to prevent step-wise progression of valvular disease.

Seronegative Spondylo- arthropathy

- **Spondyloarthropathy overview**
- **Ankylosing spondylitis**
- **Reactive arthritis**
- **Psoriatic arthritis**
- **Inflammatory bowel disease-associated arthritis**
- **Uveitis**
- **Behçet's disease**

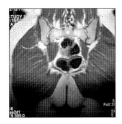
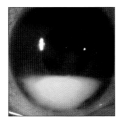
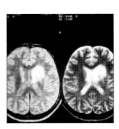
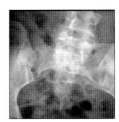

Spondyloarthropathy overview

INTRODUCTION

Spondyloarthropathies (SpAs) are a heterogeneous group of chronic inflammatory diseases of the spine. These conditions share a number of common features including:

- Sacroiliitis.
- Axial spine involvement; with or without ankylosis; with or without peripheral joint involvement.
- Seronegativity for rheumatoid factor (RF).
- Associations with HLA-B27 with familial aggregations.

Conditions that belong to the spectrum of SpAs are: 1) ankylosing spondylitis (AS); 2) reactive arthritis (ReA); 3) arthropathy of inflammatory bowel disease (IBD); 4) psoriatic arthritis (PsA); and 5) undifferentiated SpAs.

Discussed in further detail for each separate condition, the etiopathogenesis of the SpAs is largely unknown. The association between these diseases and the class I major histocompatibility (MHC) antigen HLA-B27 was first described in 1973. Infections with an unknown organism or exposure to an unknown antigen in a genetically susceptible individual, such as HLA-B27 (+), is hypothesized to result in clinical disease. This 'arthritogentic' response might involve specific microbial peptides that bind to HLA-B27 and then are presented to T cells. There may be molecular mimicry between epitopes on infecting organisms and a portion of the HLA-B27 molecule. Endogenous HLA-B27 could be antigenic resulting in autoimmunity. HLA-B27 may act in the thymus to select a repertoire of T cells that are involved in the arthritogentic response to certain infectious antigens, or HLA-B27 may be in linkage disequilibrium with a different gene responsible for disease susceptibility.

The true prevalence of the SpAs remains unclear and likely varies across populations and depends on the specific disease in the subset, such as AS or the inflammatory bowel-related SpA.

Generally, there is an increased male to female ratio of approximately 2–3:1.

Important considerations in the clinical evaluation in patients with suspected SpA include the presence of:

- Inflammatory low back pain with morning stiffness lasting greater than 1 hour; worse with prolonged rest and improved with activity.
- Oligoarthritis, distal interphlangeal (DIP) joint arthritis, and/or 'sausage digits' related to dactylitis.
- Tendonitis and/or enthesitis of the heels or Achilles tendons.
- Uveitis, often in the anterior chamber.
- Costochondritis.
- History of ulcerative colitis, Crohn's disease, or psoriasis or signs/symptoms which may be related to an undiagnosed condition.
- Recent infection of the gastrointestinal or genitourinary tract.
- History of chronic genitourinary complaints without an infectious etiology.
- Age of onset which is often less than 40 years.
- Family history to include first- and second-degree relatives with AS, psoriasis, acute uveitis, ReA, or IBD.

Keys to diagnosing SpA are obtaining a history and performing a comprehensive physical examination followed by appropriate laboratory and imaging assessment (**65–68**). The SpAs may be distinguished from each other by the extent of erosions and bone proliferation along with their distribution and symmetry (*Table 17 overleaf*). An anteroposterior projection of the pelvis with a Ferguson view using conventional radiography is often sufficient and allows for adequate evaluation of the sacroiliac joints. In early disease, when the plain radiograph may be normal, options for further analysis include computed tomography (CT), dual-energy X-ray absorptiometry bone scan (DXA), and magnetic resonance imaging (MRI) which is an excellent imaging technique to evaluate inflammation (**65**).

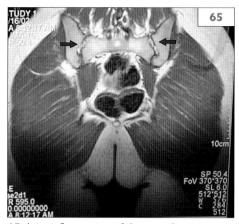

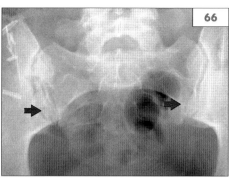

65 Joint inflammation of the sacroiliac joints on MRI scanning manifested by high intensity on this sequence (arrows). (Courtesy of Dr GF Moore.)

66 Changes in the inferior portion of the sacroiliac joints with irregularity and indistinct margins along with pseudo-widening – findings most prominent in the bottom one-third of joint (arrows). The changes are related to erosive changes of the joint. (Courtesy of Dr GF Moore.)

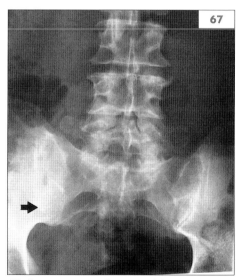

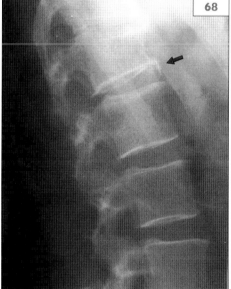

67 Asymmetric involvement of the sacroiliac (SI) joints which is more commonly seen in reactive arthritis and psoriatic arthritis (fusion or near fusion of right SI joint with relatively well preserved left SI joint, arrow). (Courtesy of Dr GF Moore.)

68 Asymmetric syndesmophytes (arrow) with nonsequential involvement of the vertebral bodies. (Courtesy of Dr GF Moore.)

New classification criteria for axial and peripheral SpA have been developed. The criteria for axial SpA have been validated and approved (*Table 18*).

Table 18 Assessment in Spondylo-Arthritis International Society (ASAS) criteria for axial spondyloarthropathy (SpA)

In patients with ≥3 months back pain and age of onset ≤45 years of age

AND

Sacroiliitis on imaging* plus ≥1 SpA feature** OR HLA-B27 plus ≥2 SpA features**

*Active (acute) inflammation on MRI highly suggestive of sacroiliitis associated with SpA, or definite radiographic sacroiliitis according to modified New York Criteria.

**SpA features: Inflammatory back pain, arthritis, enthesitis of the heal, uveitis, dactylitis, psoriasis, Crohn's or colitis, good response to NSAIDs, family history of SpA, HLA-B27, elevated CRP

CRP: C-reactive protien; MRI: magnetic resonance imaging; NSAID: nonsteroidal anti-inflammatory drug.

Table 17 Radiographic features of the subsets of the spondyloarthropathies.

Ankylosing spondylitis

The sacroiliac joints are frequently the first to show radiographic abnormalities

Erosions involve the synovial-lined inferior two-thirds of the sacroiliac joint and the involvement is often bilateral; early findings may be that of 'pseudo-widening' (**66**)

Involvement of the spine is usually in an ascending fashion without skipping segments; syndesmophytes are often thin, marginal and delicate; inflammation of the annulus fibrosis leads to 'shiny corners' and vertebral squaring (see Ankylosing spondylitis section, **75**).

Fusion of the apophyseal joints and calcification of the spinal ligaments along with bilateral syndesmophytes can cause fusion of the vertebral column resulting in the appearance of a 'bamboo spine' (see Ankylosing spondylitis section, **73, 74**).

Peripheral involvement is often in the joints closest to the spine to include the shoulders and hips

Inflammatory bowel-related spondyloarthropathies

Findings are similar to ankylosing spondylitis

Reactive arthritis

Sacroiliac involvement is often asymmetric and may be unilateral (**67**)

Involvement of the spine may have 'skip lesions' and the syndesmophytes are asymmetric and nonmarginal, with a 'jug handle' appearance (**68**)

Peripheral involvement is often in the foot with periostitis and enthesitis

Psoriatic arthritis

Spinal involvement is often similar to reactive arthritis

Approximately 95% have peripheral joint involvement which is usually asymmetric and oligoarticular affecting the distal and proximal interphlangeal joints of the hands and feet; in small joints of hands may see classic 'pencil-in-cup' deformities; (See Psoriatic arthritis section, **81, 82**); distal interphalangeal involvement is considered classic and is associated with nail involvement

Ankylosing spondylitis

DEFINITION
Ankylosing spondylitis (AS) is a chronic inflammatory disease of the axial skeleton associated with arthritis (both axial and peripheral), enthesitis, and select extraskeletal manifestations and is part of the axial spondyloarthritis disease spectrum.

EPIDEMIOLOGY AND ETIOLOGY
AS typically affects young adults with a peak age of onset between 20 and 30 years. Although historically much more common in men than women, recent estimates suggest AS has a male to female ratio of 2–3:1 and overall incidence of 7.3/100 000 person-years with prevalence ranging between 0.2% and 1.2%. AS demonstrates familial aggregation and is associated with HLA-B27 which is positive in 90–95% of Caucasians, but only 50% of African-Americans with the disease. With the prevalence of AS paralleling the frequency of HLA-B27 in the population, AS is uncommon in African blacks and Japanese where the prevalence of HLA-B27 is <1%. HLA-B27-positive adults with a disease-associated subtype have a 1–2% risk of developing AS; HLA-B27-positive first-degree relatives of patients with AS have a 10–30% risk for developing disease themselves. Other genetic and environmental factors also contribute to the risk of developing AS, with twin studies revealing disease concordance in 75% of monozygotic twins and 13% of fraternal twins.

PATHOGENESIS
Understanding of the pathogenesis of AS is limited. HLA class I molecules bind peptides from intracellular proteolysis and present them to cytotoxic T cells where glutamine interacts in the HLA-B27 B pocket with arginine, causing the B pocket to bind arthritogenic peptides. Theoretically, cytotoxic T cell autoreactivity may be induced by B27 through bacterial infection, resulting in the breakdown of peptides with bacterial and self (arthritogenic) peptides presented to cytotoxic T cells ('molecular mimicry'). An alternative theory includes protein misfolding of HLA-B27 with accumulation of unfolded protein in the endoplasmic reticulum with resultant activation of genes which activate inflammatory cytokines.

CLINICAL HISTORY
Patients present with an history of insidious onset and progression of poorly localized, chronic, inflammatory, low back pain. Characteristics useful in differentiating inflammatory from mechanical back pain include onset of back discomfort before the age of 40 years, lack of improvement with rest, improvement with exercise, and pain at night (with improvement upon arising).

A thorough medical history should attempt to identify antecedent infectious illnesses, symptoms of inflammatory bowel disease, or psoriasis. In patients with suspected AS, symptoms suggestive of extraskeletal manifestations should be sought, including aortic insufficiency (dyspnea, weight gain, and so on), inflammatory eye disease or uveitis (red or painful eye, visual deficits), cardiac conduction deficits (dyspnea or palpitations), and apical pulmonary fibrosis (dyspnea).

Low back pain is generally unilateral in early disease and becomes bilateral.

Morning stiffness is improved with activity and exacerbated with rest (so-called 'gelling phenomenon'). Enthesitis, inflammation at the area of insertion of tendon (Achilles tendon insertion), ligament, capsule or fascia (plantar fascia) into bone is common.

Peripheral joint involvement occurs in up to 70%, is asymmetric, occurs most commonly in the proximal joints (hips, shoulders) followed by the large joints of the lower extremities and is nonerosive. Hip and shoulder involvement may be the first sign of disease, with hip disease often occurring early or not at all.

Patients may complain of sleep disturbance due to pain with resultant daytime fatigue. Cervical spine involvement occurs later in the course of AS and manifests as pain and decreased range of motion (ROM). Chest expansion may be decreased due to costovertebral and costosternal enthesitis, and inflammation of the sternoclavicular joints or the manubriosternal junction may result in chest pain.

PHYSICAL EXAMINATION
AS is generally diagnosed using the modified New York criteria, with patients meeting the ASAS classification criteria for axial SpA, including both patients with AS as well as those who would be classified as nonradiographic axial SpA.

A complete joint examination should be performed to evaluate for synovitis and/or enthesitis in peripheral joints. Tenderness in the region of the sacroiliac joints or buttock may be seen with direct pressure over the sacroiliac joints (**69**) or with the patient supine, placing one of the patient's legs into the 'figure 4' position with downward pressure applied by the examiner to the flexed knee and contralateral anterior superior iliac spine. The presence of limited spinal and/or chest mobility is suggestive of AS and should be documented quantitatively to provide a baseline from which to monitor progress. Assessment of spinal mobility has traditionally been done using the Schöber (**70**) or modified Schöber test.

The four point examination (**71**) is a method for monitoring posture. Increasing occiput to wall distance (**72**) is associated with loss of lumbar and cervical lordosis and increasing thoracic spinal kyphosis.

Chest expansion is measured at the level of the fourth intercostal space or just below the breasts in females. Patients should have their arms elevated above them and hands folded behind the head. The patient is instructed to exert a maximal forced expiration followed by a maximal inspiration; expansion of less than 2.5 cm is abnormal.

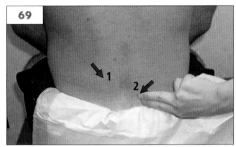

69 Tenderness over the sacroiliac joints may be observed in patients with active sacroiliitis. 1; posterior superior iliac spine. 2; SI joint. (Courtesy of Dr GF Moore.)

Table 19 ASAS Classification Criteria for axial spondyloarthritis

In patients with ≥3 months back pain and age at onset <45 years:		
Sacroiliitis on imaging **plus** ≥1 SpA feature	**OR**	**HLA-B27** **plus** ≥2 other SpA features
SpA features: • Inflammatory back pain • Arthritis • Enthesitis (heel) • Dactylitis • Psoriasis • Crohn's/colitis • Good response to NSAIDs • Family history for SpA • HLA-B27 • Elevated CRP		Sacroiliitis on imaging: • Active (acute) inflammation on MRI highly suggestive of sacroiliitis associated with SpA • Definite radiographic sacroiliitis according to modified NY criteria

CRP: C-reactive protein; MRI: magnetic resonance imaging; NSAID: nonsteroidal anti-inflammatory drugs; NY: New York; SpA: spondyloarthropathy.
(Adapted from Rudwaleit M, van der Heijde D, Landewé R, *et al.* 2009. The development of Assessment of SpondyloArthritis International Society classification criteria for axial spondyloarthritis (part II): validation and final selection. *Ann Rheum Dis* **68**:777–783, with permission.)

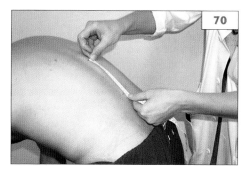

70 Schober test: 1) A mark is placed over the spinal column at a line that connects the posterior iliac spines; 2) Measure 10 cm caudally; 3) The patient bends forward as much as possible. With a normal examination, individuals will increase the distance between the two marks by at least 3–5 cm. The modified Schober test differs in that a second mark is made 5 cm below the first with the distance between the upper and lower marks measured. People with normal spinal mobility have an increase in the measured distance for the modified Schober test by at least 5 cm. (Courtesy of Dr GF Moore.)

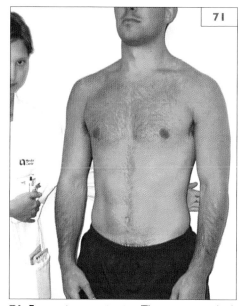

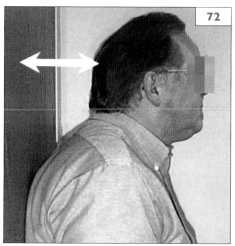

71 Four point examination: The patient is asked to stand facing away from a wall while touching their 1) occiput, 2) shoulder blades, 3) buttocks, and 4) heels against the wall. With normal lumbar lordosis, the examiner's hand should easily pass between the lumbar area and the wall. (Courtesy of Dr GF Moore.)

72 Occiput-to-wall distance is measured by asking the patient to stand with their feet against the wall; they are then asked to place their head as close to the wall as possible with the remaining distance between the occiput and wall measured. (Courtesy of Dr GF Moore.)

Confirmation of diagnosis is made by visualization of consistent radiographic findings (73–75). In cases of severe extraskeletal involvement, auscultation may reveal apical rales (with pulmonary fibrosis) or a diastolic murmur (with aortic insufficiency). Uveitis may cause scleral injection, decreased visual acuity, photophobia, and papillary miosis.

DIFFERENTIAL DIAGNOSIS

Other SpAs including ReA, PsA, and SpA associated with inflammatory bowel disease are similar and will be discussed separately. Diffuse idiopathic skeletal hyperostosis (DISH) may be confused with AS, although DISH most often represents an incidental radiographic finding (76). Sacroiliac (SI) joints in DISH are spared and the apophyseal joints are not ankylosed. Rheumatoid arthritis (RA) is differentiated from AS since it predominantly affects small peripheral joints in a symmetric pattern, and is often RF or anti-cyclic citrullinated peptide antibody (anti-CCP) positive. Fibromyalgia may also present with back pain; however, laboratory evaluation and imaging will be normal.

INVESTIGATIONS

Laboratory abnormalities in AS are typically nonspecific. Inflammatory markers are elevated in approximately 70% of patients; however, this may not correlate with disease activity. Alkaline phosphatase and serum immunoglobulin (Ig) A may be elevated but are not useful in diagnosis or following disease activity. Antinuclear antibody (ANA), RF, and anti-CCP are negative, and complement levels are normal. Due to its high prevalence, HLA-B27 is not a useful screening test in the general population. However, among individuals under the age of 45 with chronic back pain for ≥3 months, HLA-B27 testing may be a valuable tool. Additionally, in patients with acute anterior uveitis, HLA-B27-positive individuals are highly likely to have an associated SpA, with up to 90% of patients with HLA-B27-associated acute anterior uveitis having possible or definite AS.

Plain radiography is useful in diagnosis. Anterior–posterior and Ferguson's views of the pelvis should be obtained for evaluation of SI joints. Radiographic findings of sacroiliitis are typically symmetric with the earliest changes

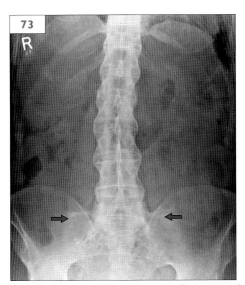 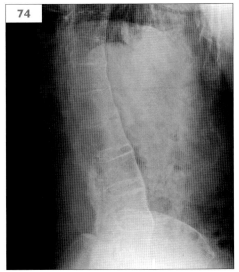

73, 74 Characteristic radiographic findings in advanced ankylosing spondylitis. Note complete fusion of the sacroiliac joints (arrows) and bridging syndesmophytes in the spine creating the appearance of a 'bamboo spine'. (Courtesy of Dr GF Moore.)

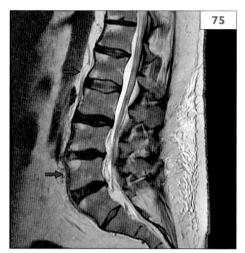

75 MRI in lower panel showing areas of inflammation (shiny corners) characteristic of AS. (Courtesy of Dr GF Moore.)

occurring in the lower third of the joint on the iliac side. Later in the course of AS, pseudowidening and then sclerosis of the SI joints occurs. Vertebral column lesions include marginal erosive lesions, bone resorption which is seen as 'shiny' squaring of the vertebral corners (77), and syndesmophytes occurring later in disease. Plain radiographs may not detect sacroiliitis in early disease or in adolescents. While no formal recommendations exist for use of CT or MRI imaging, they may be useful in patients for whom plain radiography is unrevealing, yet high clinical suspicion remains.

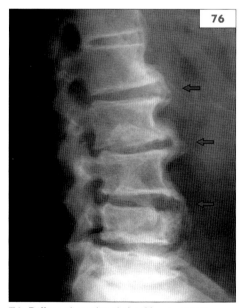

76 Diffuse idiopathic skeletal hyperostosis (DISH) may be confused with anklyosing spondylitis. Note flowing ossification of anterior longitudinal ligament (arrows); pelvic views (not shown) would show no evidence of sacroiliac involvement.

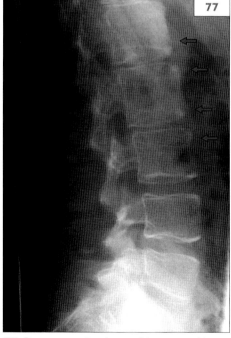

77 Bone resorption (arrows) is seen as shiny squaring of the vertebral corners, known as 'shiny corners'. (Courtesy of Dr GF Moore.)

HISTOLOGY

In sacroiliitis, inflammation initially attacks the synovium and subchondral bone with trabecular bone ultimately replacing the joint, resulting in bony ankylosis. Enthesitis occurs with initial inflammation in subchondral bone marrow and erosions, followed by healing and new bone formation which fills the erosive defects and joins the ligament as a new enthesis. In this way, spinal fusion occurs due to development of cartilage and then bone bridging the joints, termed syndesmophytes. There is a predilection for fibrocartilaginous sites and fibrous scarring may occur in intervertebral discs, at the root of aorta, through the aortic and mitral valves, and along the interventricular septum.

PROGNOSIS

The course of AS is variable and characterized by spontaneous remissions and disease flares. Overall, the prognosis is considered to be favorable with the disease running a mild or self-limited course in some individuals; however, functional limitations which increase with disease duration may be significant. Work disability is higher in those with peripheral joint involvement, especially of the hip, and has been reported in up to 30% after 10 years of disease, after which time life expectancy is also reduced. While therapies are currently available to modify disease activity in AS, complete disease control with prevention of structural damage has not been demonstrated.

Extraskeletal manifestations are associated with a worse prognosis. AS carries a 25–40% lifetime risk of acute anterior uveitis which is generally unilateral and recurrent. Cardiac complications such as inflammation and fibrosis at the aortic root, aortic insufficiency, and conduction system defects such as complete heart block are possible. Pulmonary complications may present as cough, dyspnea, or hemoptysis and include chest wall rigidity and restricted pulmonary function tests (PFTs) with apical fibrobullous disease a late manifestation. AS may indirectly affect the kidneys through secondary amyloidosis, IgA nephropathy, or through chronic nonsteroidal anti-inflammatory drug (NSAID) use. Osteoporosis is often evident early in the disease course and the combination of an ankylosed spine and osteoporosis increases the risk of spinal fracture. Rare neurologic complications include cauda equina and atlantoaxial subluxation.

MANAGEMENT

Physical therapy and exercise are the cornerstones of therapy in AS with some patients responding well to exercise alone. Scheduled NSAIDs should be used as first-line therapy and can significantly reduce inflammatory back pain and radiographic progression of AS. Antitumor necrosis factor (anti-TNF) agents have efficacy in treating the skeletal manifestations of AS and attenuate bony destruction. Uveitis requires prompt attention with topical steroids and mydriatics. Delayed treatment for uveitis may lead to synechiae and glaucoma. If systemic therapy is required for uveitis, TNF inhibition with a monoclonal antibody is recommended. Traditional disease-modifying, antirheumatic drugs (DMARDs), such as sulfasalazine (SSZ), may be of benefit in treatment of peripheral arthritis, but axial symptoms are generally unresponsive. Methotrexate (MTX) and leflunomide may also be useful in the treatment of peripheral arthritis; however, few data are currently available on either of these agents. There is a limited role for systemic corticosteroids in AS, but these may be useful topically for treatment of uveitis and for local intra-articular treatment.

Reactive arthritis

DEFINITION
Reactive arthritis (ReA) is a form of seronegative SpA that is induced by select infections and which manifests as a systemic illness characterized primarily by an inflammatory synovitis from which viable organisms cannot be cultured.

EPIDEMIOLOGY AND ETIOLOGY
ReA incidence is estimated to be 10–30 per 100 000 person-years with a total prevalence of less than 1 per 10 000 people. ReA is more common in men than women with peak incidence in younger men between the ages of 20 to 40 years. Approximately 50% of ReA cases are attributable to a specific pathogen, typically those associated with urethritis or dysentery (*Chlamydia, Salmonella, Shigella, Yersenia*, and *Campylobacter* spp.).

PATHOGENESIS
Triggering pathogens in ReA are most often gram-negative obligate or facultative, intracellular aerobic pathogens with a lipopolysaccharide (LPS)-containing outer membrane. The organisms are invasive and in some cases disseminate from the mucosa to the joints. Bacterial antigens have been isolated in joints in ReA, but the significance of this finding is not clear. Although the presence of HLA B27 is not required for the development of ReA (seen in ~50% of cases), its presence is associated with disease chronicity. Although ReA pathologenesis is not completely understood, it has been speculated that the presentation of unknown bacterial antigens (or self antigens) via HLA B27 to cytotoxic T cells plays a central role in chronic inflammation characteristic of ReA.

CLINICAL HISTORY AND PHYSICAL EXAMINATION
Usually there is a lag of 1–4 weeks between infection (often asymptomatic) and musculoskeletal complaints in ReA. The musculoskeletal presentation can be of an acute nature and may mimic septic arthritis. Joint involvement is typically asymmetric, oligoarticular, and often confined to the knees, ankles, and feet. Chest pain caused by costochondritis is not uncommon. Enthesitis (inflammation at tendon insertions) is characteristic, with Achilles tendonitis and plantar fasciitis being the most common. Dactylitis (a 'sausage digit') which results from joint swelling and tendon inflammation is characteristic of ReA. Low back pain and stiffness lasting greater than 1 hour is often present and may be due to sacroiliitis. Extra-articular manifestations include:
- Keratoderma blenorrhagicum (**78**): Papulosquamous rash resembling pustular psoriasis, affecting the palms and soles.

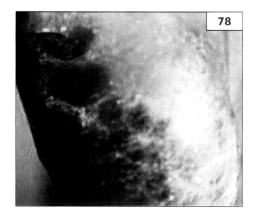

78 Keratoderma blenorrhagicum characteristic of reactive arthritis is a 'psoriatic like' process often found on the soles of the feet. (Courtesy of Dr GF Moore.)

- Circinate balanitis (**79**): Plaque-like, hyperkeratotic lesions on the penis, associated with urogenital ReA; these resolve spontaneously.
- Dysuria and/or urethritis: May be associated with genitourinary-induced disease and may be infectious but can also be noninfectious and seen with ReA following dysentery.
- Painless oral ulcers.
- Hyperkeratotic nails.
- Uveitis and sterile conjunctivitis (**80**): Ocular injection/inflammation mandate prompt ophthalmology referral.

DIFFERENTIAL DIAGNOSIS

The differential diagnosis in ReA includes septic arthritis (including that from gonococcal infection), Lyme disease, rheumatic fever, PsA, and inflammatory bowel-related arthritis. Other entities to consider include gout (typically affecting older patients) and RA (more common in women and more often characterized by symmetric and polyarticular presentation compared to ReA).

INVESTIGATIONS

The diagnosis of ReA is based on clinical grounds. As a form of seronegative arthritis, RF and ANA are almost universally negative. Assessing HLA B27 status is of little or no clinical utility. Complete blood count may show leukocytosis, elevated platelet count, and a normocytic or microcytic anemia reflective of anemia of chronic inflammation. Although nonspecific, erythrocyte sedimentation rate (ESR) and C-reactive protein (CRP) are often elevated. Synovial fluid analysis typically demonstrates inflammatory joint fluid (5000–50 000 cells/mm^3 with predominance of polymorphonuclear cells [PMNs]). Synovial fluid cultures are typically negative. Stool cultures and urogenital cultures should be obtained to evaluate for causative infections. Because ReA may be the initial manifestation of human immunodeficiency virus (HIV), appropriate testing should be completed in at-risk patients.

In chronic ReA, radiographs may demonstrate characteristic findings in the spine and the peripheral joints. In the sacroiliac joints, findings are often asymmetric and include erosions and ankylosis. In the spine, findings include large nonmarginal syndesmophytes (**68**). Only 25% of patients with ReA develop sacroiliac changes. Radiographs of involved joints may demonstrate evidence of enthesitis and periostitis, along with erosions of the proximal interphalangeal (PIP) or, less commonly, the DIP joints, especially of the toes.

HISTOLOGY

As previously noted, synovial fluid analysis in ReA demonstrates a moderately inflamed fluid with cell counts of 5000–50 000 cell/mm^3 with a predominance of PMNs (although in later stages there may be increased expression of lymphocytes and monocytes). Large vacuolar macrophages containing intact lymphocytes or fragmented nuclei may be seen on synovianalysis, though their presence is nondiagnostic. Although rarely performed, biopsy of involved synovium shows nonspecific changes of chronic inflammation.

PROGNOSIS

The prognosis is variable for patients with ReA, though most patients (~70–80%) will recover fully over many weeks to months. A significant proportion of patients will experience relapse if they should develop another gastrointestinal or genitourinary infection. Approximately 20–30% of patients will develop a chronic form of ReA with peripheral and/or axial involvement.

MANAGEMENT

Principles of ReA management include:
- Treatment of the triggering infection event.
- NSAIDs are often used first-line in the treatment of musculoskeletal symptoms.
- Refractory or severe disease may require either oral or intra-articular corticosteroids (although response to these agents may be blunted compared to other conditions).

- DMARDs, often SSZ, may be used with a more protracted disease course; other DMARDs used include MTX, azathioprine (AZA), leflunomide, and biologic agents targeting TNF (e.g. etanercept, infliximab, and adalimumab).
- Doxycycline may have a treatment role, especially in genitourinary-induced ReA; combination antibiotic therapy with doxycycline and rifampin may be superior to doxycycline alone.

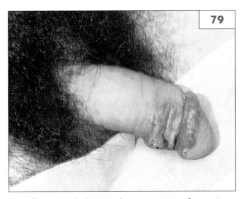

79 Circinate balanitis characteristic of reactive arthritis is a 'psoriatic-like' lesion found on the shaft of the penis or on the glans. (Courtesy of Dr GF Moore.)

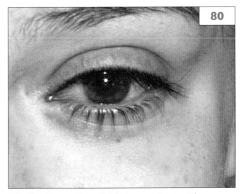

80 Sterile conjunctivitis in a patient with reactive arthritis. (Courtesy of Dr GF Moore.)

Psoriatic arthritis

DEFINITION

Psoriatic arthritis (PsA) is a systemic inflammatory arthritis, characterized by inflammation of peripheral joints, spinal inflammation, dactylitis, and enthesitis that occurs in the context of psoriatic skin disease.

EPIDEMIOLOGY AND ETIOLOGY

PsA affects men and women equally and its onset peaks in the 20s to 30s. Psoriasis affects 2% of the population, and PsA co-exists in approximately 25% of psoriasis patients. In approximately 10–15% of PsA patients, the onset of the inflammatory arthritis may precede the development of psoriatic skin disease.

Environmental, infectious, and genetic factors have been implicated in the pathogenesis of PsA. Streptococcal infections have been reported to precede the onset of guttate psoriasis, but definitive evidence for an infectious trigger for either psoriasis or PsA is lacking. Occasionally, trauma to a certain joint may be temporally associated with the onset of a systemic inflammatory arthritis, a process known as the 'deep Koebner phenomenon.' The HLA-CW6 allele has been associated with psoriasis and, to a lesser extent, with PsA. The HLA-B27 allele is associated with spinal involvement in patients with PsA. TNF-α polymorphisms have also been implicated in the development of PsA.

CLINICAL HISTORY AND PHYSICAL EXAMINATION

The presenting symptoms of PsA are variable, but similar to the other spondyloarthritides, and may include:
- Peripheral joint inflammation leading to joint swelling, stiffness, and pain.
- Dactylitis or 'sausage digit' (**81**).
- Inflammation at areas of tendon attachment (enthesitis; e.g. achilles tendonitis or plantar fasciitis).
- Inflammation of the axial spine leading to pain and marked morning stiffness in addition to stiffness following periods of prolonged rest; this may be associated with sacroiliitis (more likely to be unilateral than in AS).

Most patients present with an oligoarthritis or a polyarthritis (the latter can closely resemble RA), and the onset of symptoms is usually insidious. The small joints of the hands and feet are most commonly involved, and unlike RA, the DIP joints are frequently involved (one-third of patients) (**82**). Morning stiffness, pain and swelling may be present. Five clinical patterns of PsA have been described:
- Asymmetric oligoarthritis.
- Symmetric polyarthritis.
- Predominant DIP involvement.
- Spondyloarthritis.
- Arthritis mutilans.

Extra-articular features are common (**83, 84**), and include skin psoriasis, dystrophic nail changes, and inflammatory eye disease. Eye disease (e.g. uveitis) is seen in 7–18% of patients and is more common in those with spinal involvement. Nail disease is seen in two-thirds of patients and includes pitting and ridging of the nails and onycholysis. Nail disease correlates with involvement of the DIP joints (**82**).

DIFFERENTIAL DIAGNOSIS

Differential diagnosis includes RA, osteoarthritis (OA), ReA, AS, septic arthritis, gout, calcium pyrophosphate dehydrate (pseudogout) (CPPD) arthropathy, and enteropathic arthritis. Other causes of marked DIP joint arthritis include generalized OA and the rare disorder, multicentric reticulohistiocytosis.

INVESTIGATIONS

There is no laboratory test which is diagnostic for psoriatic arthritis. RF is generally not present, but may be seen in low titers in a minority of patients. Anticitrullinated peptide antibodies (anti-CCP) are found in approximately 5% of patients, generally those with a symmetric polyarthritis. Inflammatory markers, including the ESR and CRP, may be elevated (especially in polyarticular disease) but generally to a lesser extent than in RA. Hyperuricemia is common, owing to increased cell turnover (and co-existent gout can be seen). Complement levels are generally normal or elevated. Synovial fluid analysis generally demonstrates a sterile, inflammatory infiltrate with neutrophil predominance. Synovial fluid white blood cell (WBC) counts are typically

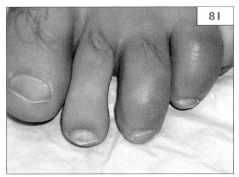

81 Dactylitis of the third and fourth digits of the left foot. (Courtesy of Dr GF Moore.)

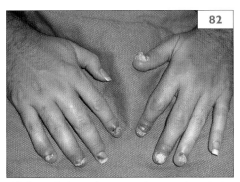

82 Interphalangeal joint involvement is typical for psoriatic arthritis; note that this patient also has nail changes with associated distal interphalangeal joint synovitis. (Courtesy of Dr GF Moore.)

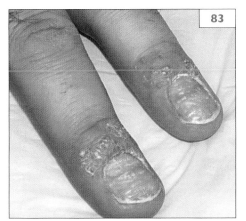

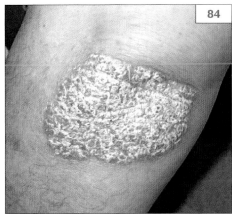

83, 84 Extra-articular manifestations of psoriatic arthritis. 83: Nail pitting and dystrophic nail changes; 84: typical appearance of plaque psoriasis. (Courtesy of Dr GF Moore.)

>1000–2000 cells/mm^3 but usually less than 25 000 cells/mm^3. Radiographic features may include asymmetric joint involvement, involvement of interphalangeal joints of fingers and toes, features of bony resorption or erosion (when advanced may lead to 'pencil-in-cup' deformity), joint space narrowing, enthesophytes, periosteitis, and sacroiliitis. Bone mineralization is generally preserved (**85, 86**). Spine films may show evidence of spondyloarthritis or sacroiliitis, the latter may present with asymmetric involvement (**87**).

HISTOLOGY

The synovium in PsA is typically more vascular than that of RA, but contains few monocytes and macrophages and is less hyperplastic. Vascular endothelial growth factor (VEGF) is richly expressed in the synovium in PsA. TNF-α is highly expressed in PsA in both the skin and joint lesions. The natural history of PsA is variable from patient to patient and can range from episodic mild flares to a progressive, destructive chronic arthritis.

PROGNOSIS

There is little correlation between the severity and activity of the skin and joint manifestations in PsA. Elevated inflammatory markers are a poor prognostic feature in polyarticular disease. Patients with PsA have increased mortality relative to the general population, perhaps owing to associations of systemic inflammation with cardiovascular disease burden. Poor prognostic features in PsA include polyarticular disease, poor response to initial therapies, young age at onset, acute onset, elevated inflammatory markers, and previous glucocorticoid (GC) use.

MANAGEMENT

First-line treatment for PsA generally consists of NSAIDs. GCs may be effective, but are reported to exacerbate skin disease; intra-articular GC has proven to be a useful adjunct.

Systemic immunomodulatory therapy is indicated if three or more joints remain inflamed despite conventional therapies, or for resistant axial, entheseal, or dactylitic disease. Systemic therapy may also be indicated for the management of severe skin disease, even when arthritic symptoms are mild.

SSZ has the best evidence for efficacy in PsA, but does not benefit skin or axial disease. MTX (weekly dosing) is widely used, despite having few trial data supporting its benefit, and may be helpful in the management of both peripheral and axial joint disease, as well as the skin. Cyclosporine is effective but its use is limited by its toxicities (primarily renal insufficiency and hypertension).

Leflunomide is also useful in managing both skin and arthritic manifestations. TNF-α inhibitors have proven to be quite effective in controlling peripheral and axial arthritis and retarding radiographic progression, as well as improving skin, entheseal, and dactylitic disease.

There are few data regarding the use of combination therapies for the management of PsA, although this strategy may be effective in select patients. Other biologic therapies, such as the inhibition of T cell co-stimulation or inhibition of interleukin (IL)-12/23 may prove to be useful in the management of PsA, but are considered investigational therapies at this time.

85 Radiographs demonstrating severe destructive changes of psoriatic arthritis (so-called arthritis mutilans). Note the ankylosis of the left fourth distal interphalangeal joint, the pencil-in-cup deformity developing at the left first metacarpal phalangeal joint and the advanced destructive changes at multiple other small joints, with overall preservation of bone mineralization. (Courtesy of Dr GF Moore.)

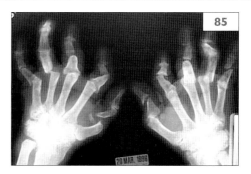

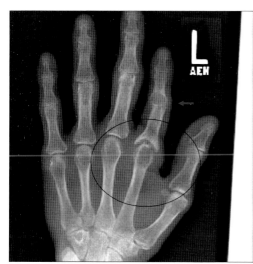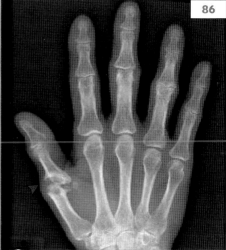

86 Radiographs of a psoriatic arthritis patient showing development of pencil-in-cup deformity (circle) at the left second metacarpal–phalangeal (MCP) joint, ankylosis of the left second proximal interphalangeal joint (arrow), and destruction of the right first MCP joint (arrowhead), with preservation of bone mineralization. Note the asymmetric involvement of psoriatic arthritis. (Courtesy of Dr GF Moore.)

87 Anterior–posterior radiograph of the pelvis in a patient with psoriatic arthritis and inflammatory low back pain; findings demonstrate joint space widening and sclerosis of the right sacroiliac joint (arrow).

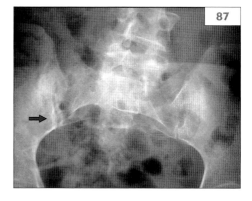

Inflammatory bowel disease-associated arthritis

DEFINITION
Inflammatory arthritis is a well-recognized, extra-intestinal manifestation of inflammatory bowel disease (IBD; most commonly Crohn's disease or ulcerative colitis). The arthritis of IBD shares similarities with the other seronegative spondyloarthritides as it may present with enthesitis, sacroiliitis spondylitis, or peripheral arthritis.

EPIDEMIOLOGY AND ETIOLOGY
Approximately one-quarter of IBD patients will report arthralgias, and the incidence of overt arthritis ranges from approximately 10% to 20%. IBD-related arthropathy frequently occurs in patients with other extraintestinal manifestations of IBD, including pyoderma gangrenosum, erythema nodosum, stomatitis, uveitis, fistula formation, and others (**88**). The arthritis may precede the diagnosis of IBD. Often these patients will be classified as an undifferentiated SpA until the bowel symptoms manifest. There is a significant overlap between AS and IBD-related arthritis. Up to 60% of AS patients have subclinical inflammatory changes in the small or large intestines suggestive of subclinical IBD. Pediatric and adult IBD patients may exhibit arthritic symptoms and both sexes are affected equally. Similar to the other spondyloarthritides, HLA-B27 is associated with IBD-associated arthritides, especially those with axial involvement. However, HLA-B27 is not associated with type II arthropathy (see below), which associates with the HLA-B44 haplotype.

PATHOGENESIS
The pathogenesis of IBD-related arthritis is incompletely understood. However, several observations have been made which may help describe the sequence of events leading to the development of the arthritis symptoms. Patients with IBD have a diminished capacity to defend against gut bacteria. It has been proposed that intestinal infection with a select micro-organism in a genetically susceptible host leads to further inflammation in gut mucosa, initiating an inflammatory cascade with activation of T lymphocytes with circulating immune complexes and memory T cells localizing to the joints and causing synovitis.

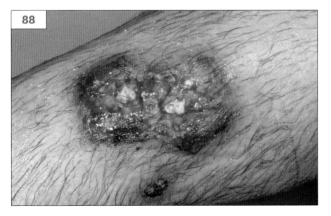

88 A patient with newly diagnosed Crohn's disease manifesting with polyarthralgias and pyoderma gangrenosum.

CLINICAL HISTORY AND PHYSICAL EXAMINATION

The arthritis of IBD may affect the axial or appendicular skeleton and may cause entheseal inflammation. Patients may present with spondylitis, sacroiliitis, enthesitis, arthritis of the peripheral joints, or a combination thereof. Spondylitis and sacroiliitis typically manifest with inflammatory back pain and associated stiffness that is worse in the morning and exacerbated by prolonged periods of rest. The peripheral arthritis tends to correlate with the activity of the bowel disease in ulcerative colitis, but not that of Crohn's disease. Two patterns of peripheral arthritis in IBD have been recognized (*Table 20*).

Spondylitis occurs in up to 25% of IBD patients but is often subclinical. Men are affected by spondylitis more frequently than women. The spondylitis does not typically correlate with the degree of intestinal inflammation. Sacroiliitis is common though often asymptomatic. Similar to IBD-related spondylitis, sacroiliitis may not correlate with activity of IBD. On physical examination, spondylitis may manifest by limited range of motion in the spine (abnormal Schober test or limited thoracic excursion), while sacroilitis may lead to localized tenderness over the involved joints.

DIFFERENTIAL DIAGNOSIS

The differential diagnosis for IBD is broad and depends on the clinical presentation. Given that IBD is frequently treated with immunosuppressive agents, synovial fluid analysis should be done to rule out septic arthritis in patients presenting with a mono- or oligoarthritis. Other entities which can mimic IBD-associated arthritis include Behçet's disease (BD), Whipple's disease, ReA, and celiac disease, given that all may have both musculoskeletal and gastrointestinal manifestations. In patients with known IBD, musculoskeletal manifestations may be related to treatments of their bowel disease. TNF inhibitors and other immunosuppressants which are frequently used in IBD may predispose to opportunistic infections, and have rarely been associated with the development of drug-induced lupus. Avascular necrosis may result from extended use of corticosteroids and may mimic a monoarticular arthritis is patients with IBD.

Table 20 Patterns of peripheral arthritis in inflammatory bowel disease (IBD)

Type I	Type II
Acute onset	Persistent disease course – frequent relapses
Generally self-limiting	Polyarticular involvement
Associated with flares of IBD	Frequently involves MCP joints; less commonly MTP, PIP, shoulder, wrist, elbow, and ankle joints
Oligoarticular involvement (<6 joints)	
Nondeforming	May be migratory
Occurs early in disease course	Affects 3–4% of IBD patients
Commonly affects knee	Does not typically parallel activity of bowel disease
Affects 5% of IBD patients	

MCP: metacarpal–phalangeal; MTP: metatarsal–phalangeal; PIP: proximal interphalangeal.

INVESTIGATIONS

No single laboratory abnormality is unique to IBD-associated arthropathy. Most investigations are performed to exclude other entities. Common to other inflammatory conditions, elevations in acute phase reactants (ESR, CRP, platelets) with associated anemia of chronic disease are frequent, but not universal. Elevated RF is generally not seen. Despite the well-described HLA associations, screening for HLA haplotypes is not routinely recommended. Synovial fluid analysis generally shows a WBC of fewer than 15 000 cells/mm^3, with PMN predominance. Radiographs of peripheral joints may demonstrate soft tissue swelling, effusion, periosteal reaction, and juxta-articular osteoporosis. Generally, IBD arthropathy is nonerosive and nondestructive. Imaging of the axial skeleton may show typical changes of AS (bridging syndesmophytes, loss of lumbar lordosis) though Romanus lesions (the so-called 'shiny corners' on vertebral bodies) are less common, whereas squaring of the vertebral bodies is more common. Sacroiliitis may be seen on plain radiography or with advanced imaging modalities (**89**). Frequently, sacroiliitis is present on CT or MRI even when a patient is asymptomatic.

HISTOLOGY

Although infrequently performed, synovial biopsy in patients with IBD-associated arthropathy demonstrates nonspecific inflammatory findings such as increased vascularity, synovial proliferation, and infiltration of PMNs.

MANAGEMENT

In many instances, effective control of the intestinal inflammation will result in control of the arthritic manifestations. However, additional agents may be necessary to control the musculoskeletal manifestations of IBD, particularly with axial involvement. Colectomy for refractory ulcerative colitis will usually resolve a peripheral arthropathy though axial symptoms may persist.

Agents used in the treatment of IBD and IBD-associated arthritis are summarized in *Table 21*.

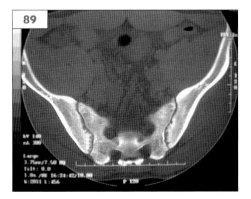

89 CT scan of the pelvis showing bilateral erosive sacroiliitis in a patient with Crohn's disease, predominantly involving iliac bone.

Several agents are effective in treating both the IBD and the associated arthropathy. Because the arthropathy of IBD is nonerosive, it is less important to initiate immunosuppressive therapies than in other inflammatory arthritides. Symptomatic control may be obtained with NSAIDs; however, they must be used with great caution secondary to their gastrointestinal side-effects. NSAIDs may be effective in managing both axial and peripheral symptoms. Sulfasalazine (SSZ) may be beneficial in the management of the peripheral arthritis but is less so for axial symptoms. Many patients with IBD are already taking SSZ (or related agent) for the treatment of their bowel disease. If the arthritic symptoms remain uncontrolled with SSZ, or if axial symptoms predominate, MTX can be added. If the toxicity profile of MTX is unacceptable, alternative agents, such as AZA or 6-mercaptopurine, may be used. Intra-articular or systemic corticosteroids may be used selectively. In patients who fail to respond to the aforementioned therapies, TNF-inhibitors may be beneficial. Of the TNF-inhibitors available, only the monoclonal antibodies (i.e. infliximab and adalimumab) appear to be effective for the treatment of IBD. The selection of immunosuppressive agents should be done in conjunction with the patient's gastroenterologist to optimize control of both bowel and musculoskeletal symptoms.

Table 21 Effects of pharmacologic agents on IBD and associated arthritis

Drug	Peripheral arthritis	Axial arthritis	Bowel disease
NSAIDs	X	X	May worsen
Systemic glucocorticoids	X	?	X
Sulfasalazine	X		X
Methotrexate	X	X	X
Azathioprine	X		X
Etanercept	X	X	
Infliximab	X	X	X
Adalimumab	X	X	X
Certolizumab pegol*	X	X	X
Golimumab*	X	X	

*Data with certolizumab pegol and golimumab in the management of IBD arthritis are limited, but have shown similar efficacy in the management of other inflammatory arthritides as other monoclonal tumor necrosis factor (TNF) inhibitors.

Uveitis

DEFINITION

Inflammation of the inner eye has been loosely characterized as uveitis. The diagnostic term uveitis indicates the presence of inflammation in the uveal tract which includes the iris, ciliary body, and choroid.

EPIDEMIOLOGY AND ETIOLOGY

Etiologies for uveitis can be categorized as infectious *vs.* noninfectious. Noninfectious causes include those associated with autoimmune diseases, trauma, malignancy-related, and chemical-induced. Approximately one-third to one-half of noninflammatory uveitis is associated with an underlying rheumatic condition, with seronegative SpA being the most common secondary rheumatic cause. A substantial proportion of uveitis cases (30–50%) are idiopathic. The classification of uveitis may be completed on the basis of pathology (HLA-B27-associated *vs.* other), etiology, and anatomic location. The location of ocular involvement is very helpful in determining the etiology and diagnosis (**90**).

Involvement of the iris (also called iritis) and/or the ciliary body (cyclitis) is referred to iridocyclitis or anterior uveitis. Inflammation in the region of the ciliary body and the vitreous with minimal changes in the anterior and posterior segments is referred to as intermediate uveitis, and inflammation limited to the vitreous is referred to as vitritis. Retinal involvement is referred to as retinitis or posterior uveitis. The term posterior uveitis also applies to inflammation of choroid. If all segments of the eye are involved, the term panuveitis is applied (**91**).

PATHOGENESIS

The pathogenesis of uveitis remains poorly understood. Like other autoimmune conditions, the immune pathogenesis of uveitis may result from an antigen-specific immune response and the subsequent expression of proinflammatory cytokines. Recent research also suggests that the disease may be associated with the activation of receptors in the innate immune system (including Toll-like receptors) by molecules such as LPS derived from gram-negative bacteria which are speculated to serve as a possible disease trigger.

CLINICAL HISTORY AND PHYSICAL EXAMINATION

Patients with uveitis present differently depending on the location of inflammation (*Table 22*). Anterior uveitis typically presents as pain, redness, and photophobia, often unilateral. Intermediate uveitis often has more of an insidious onset with floaters and haziness of vision. Posterior uveitis is also insidious with blurred vision, floaters, and scotomata. Both intermediate and posterior uveitis is relatively free of redness and pain.

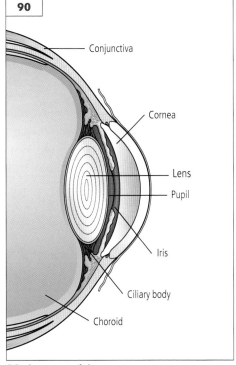

90

Conjunctiva

Cornea

Lens

Pupil

Iris

Ciliary body

Choroid

90 Anatomy of the eye.

The parameters used clinically to characterize uveitis include the anatomic location, laterality (unilateral or bilateral), acute or insidious onset and duration. Most of this information can be ascertained clinically except for the location, which is obtained via a slit lamp and dilated examination, typically by ophthalmology. Other important historical features include a past history of systemic disease, immunosuppressive therapy use, history of sexually transmitted diseases or exposure to contagions such as tuberculosis, history of arthritis particularly of the low back, oral or genital ulcerations, or diarrhea.

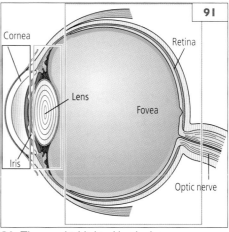

91 The area highlighted by the boxes demonstrates the varying anatomic location of uveitis including anterior (red box), intermediate (green box), and posterior (blue box) forms of uveitis. If all three areas are involved, this is classified as panuveitis.

Table 22 Clinical manifestations of uveitis based on anatomic location of involvement

Acute anterior uveitis

Inflammation of the iris and/or ciliary body

Red, painful eye

Photophobia

Blurred vision

Often unilateral

Acute onset over hours to days

Slit lamp examination may demonstrate cells in the anterior chamber with 'flare,' miosis, keratic precipitates, and hypopyon (**92**)

Intermediate uveitis

Floaters or haziness of vision

Nonpainful

Slit lamp examination may show 'snow banking'

Posterior uveitis

Blurred vision

Nonpainful

Slit lamp examination may show vitreous cells, vasculitis of the retina, vessel sheathing, or exudates

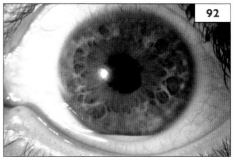

92 Layering of inflammatory debris in the anterior chamber known as hypopyon in addition to irregularly shaped pupil due to synechia between lens and iris; patient with juvenile idiopathic arthritis and uveitis. (With permission, American College of Rheumatology.)

There are several rheumatic diseases that are associated with uveitis (*Table 23*).

Uveitis in the setting of juvenile inflammatory arthritis (JIA) is usually located in the anterior chamber, but unlike other forms of anterior uveitis, is relatively asymptomatic. These patients should be screened routinely, even if asymptomatic, since progression of the condition can lead to permanent visual losses.

DIFFERENTIAL DIAGNOSIS

The differential diagnosis for all forms of uveitis, especially anterior uveitis, is broad and again is dictated by the location of anatomic involvement (*Table 24*). It is important to exclude infectious causes before initiating systemic therapy (*Table 25*). Masquerading diseases can rarely include malignancy (especially lymphoma and leukemia).

Acute anterior uveitis (AAU) in adults is frequently idiopathic, but can be HLA-B27-related. Up to 60% of patients with AAU will have an associated seronegative SpA, such as AS, PsA, arthritis secondary to IBD, or ReA.

INVESTIGATIONS

Laboratory and radiographic assessment typically includes a targeted evaluation to rule out infection or identify underlying rheumatic disease (*Table 25*). Chest radiograph (evaluating for hilar adenopathy associated with sarcoidosis), and a free treponemal antibody (FTA) screening test for syphilis are appropriate. Though the risk of tuberculosis causing uveitis is low, a purified protein derivative (PPD) is indicated in high-risk patients. ANA and RF are rarely helpful in the evaluation of uveitis. HLA-B27 testing is appropriate in the patient with AAU, but not in the individual with intermediate, posterior, or chronic disease. Depending on the clinical scenario, other laboratory and imaging testing may be appropriate.

HISTOLOGY

Ocular inflammation leads to vessel dilatation, vascular permeability, and migration of inflammatory cells. These changes ultimately lead to the physical findings of ciliary injection, aqueous flare, keratitic precipitates, hypopyon, and vitreous cells.

PROGNOSIS

The prognosis of uveitis is largely dependent on the degree of involvement and the location of involvement. Untreated or refractory uveitis can lead to blindness. Treatment, especially with immunosuppressants, can predispose to ocular infections such as fungal infections, which can be sight limiting or lead to enucleation.

MANAGEMENT

The treatment of uveitis is often determined by the location, etiology, and severity of disease.

Table 23 Rheumatic conditions associated with uveitis and clinical characteristics

Rheumatic disease	Onset	Laterality	Location
Ankylosing spondylitis	Acute	Unilateral	Anterior
JIA	Insidious	Bilateral	Anterior
Psoriatic arthritis	Acute	Inilateral	Anterior
Reactive arthritis	Acute	Unilateral	Anterior
Sarcoidosis	Variable	Variable	All chambers
Behçet's disease	Acute	Unilateral	Posterior

Important in this process is communication between the ophthalmologist and the clinician providing supportive care. Anterior uveitis is treated initially with topical therapy to include corticosteroids and mydriatics to prevent synechiae. Topical GCs, however, are associated with ocular complications to include cataracts, glaucoma, and infectious complications.

Oral or injectable corticosteroids may be added in the patient that is resistant to topical therapy or who has severe bilateral disease. In these patients, oral prednisone may also act as a bridge to immunosuppressant therapy. In addition to systemic GCs, commonly used immuno-suppressants to treat refractory or severe uveitis include MTX, AZA, cyclosporine, mycophenolate mofetil (MMF), and cyclophosphamide (CTX). In some instances, anti-TNF therapy has been used.

Table 24 Differential diagnosis of uveitis based on anatomic location of inflammation

Anterior

Young adults

HLA-B27-related

Sarcoidosis

Syphilis

Fuch's heterochromic iridocyclitis

Behçet's disease

Older adults

Idiopathic

Sarcoidosis

Masquerading syndromes

Intermediate

Pars planitis

Multiple sclerosis

Sarcoidosis

Infections to include Lyme disease, syphilis, or tuberculosis

Fuch's heterochromic iridocyclitis

Posterior

Toxoplasmosis (adults)

Lyme disease

Histoplasmosis

Panuveitis (with retinal vasculitis)

Sarcoidosis

Tuberculosis

Syphilis

Behçet's disease

Vogt–Koyanagi–Harada syndrome

Table 25 Infectious causes of uveitis

Bacterial

Mycobacteria

Syphilis

Leprosy

Brucellosis

Leptospirosis

Lyme disease

Whipple's disease

Viral

Epstein–Barr virus

Cytomeglovirus

Measles

Varicella

Herpes

Mumps

HIV

West Nile virus

Fungal

Histoplasmosis

Coccidiomycosis

Blastomycosis

Candidiasis

Aspergillosis

Cryptococcus

Parasitic

Toxoplasmosis

Acanthamoeba

Cystercercosis

Onchocerciasis

Toxocariasis

Behçet's disease

DEFINITION
Behçet's disease (BD), also known as Behçet's syndrome or Adamantiades–Behçet disease, is an inflammatory syndrome characterized by recurrent oral and genital ulcerations, eye and skin lesions, and pathergy (an exaggerated response to simple trauma).

EPIDEMIOLOGY AND ETIOLOGY
Although encountered worldwide, BD has a much higher reported prevalence in the Middle East and the Mediterranean regions (0.1% of the population of Turkey). In Northern Europe and North America, however, it is much less common. Overall, BD appears to slightly more common in men in the Middle East with a slight female predominance in North America and Northern Europe. BD commonly presents among patients in their 20s to 30s.

The cause of BD is unknown. Genetics clearly play an important role with multiple genes currently implicated. There is a strong association with the HLA B51-01 marker. It is unclear whether the HLA B51-01 gene plays a role in the pathogenesis or whether it is associated (via linkage disequilibrium) with the presence of other disease-related genes. Several different micro-organisms have been suggested to act as triggers in BD including herpes simplex virus, *Streptococcus sanguis*, *Escherichia coli*, and *Staphylococcus aureus* without definitive evidence for any single cause.

PATHOGENESIS
The pathogenesis of BD is not well understood. As with many autoimmune diseases, a popular theory suggests that an environmental trigger incites an abnormal immunological response in a genetically susceptible individual (the nature of the trigger and the genes involved are yet to be fully elicited). Subsequent to this 'inciting event,' heat shock proteins stimulate a predominant T helper type 1 (Th1) cell response through interaction with Toll-like receptors. The T lymphocytes involved have been noted to be of the $\delta\gamma$ type. The expression of inflammatory cytokines, including IL-1 and TNF-α, is increased. Effector cells, such as neutrophils and natural killer (NK) cells are likewise activated and cause tissue injury that phenotypically presents as BD.

CLINICAL HISTORY AND PHYSICAL EXAMINATION
BD has a wide clinical variability, with exacerbations and remissions often found. Multisystem involvement is common and clinical findings are presented in *Table 26*.

Table 26 Clinical findings in Behçet's disease

Skin/mucous membranes

Oral aphthous ulcers: earliest, most common manifestation, typically painful (**93**)

Genital ulcerations (**95**)

Erythema nodosum

Superficial thrombophlebitis

Papular skin lesions/acneiform-like lesions (**94**)

Pathergy: exaggerated response to minimal stimuli (i.e. papule formation 24–48 hours following routine blood draw) (**96**)

Eye

Uveitis: hypopneon uveitis classic (purulent debris in the anterior chamber) (**97**)

Retinal vasculitis

Musculoskeletal

Nondeforming, nonerosive inflammatory oligoarthritis, most commonly of large joints (**98**)

Neurologic

Central nervous system involvement rare (pyramidal, cerebellar, sphincter disturbances and behavioral changes) (**99**)

Cranial nerve involvement

Dural sinus thrombosis

Aseptic meningitis

Pulmonary

Pulmonary artery aneurysms; may present with hemoptysis; major cause of mortality (**100**, **101**)

Gastrointestinal

Abdominal pain, diarrhea and melena; due to mucosal/gastrointestinal ulcerations

Vascular

Thrombophlebitis/thrombosis of major vessels (Budd–Chiari); arterial stenoses, occlusions and aneurysms

Renal

Hematuria and/or proteinuria

Amyloidosis (late complication)

Glomerulonephritis

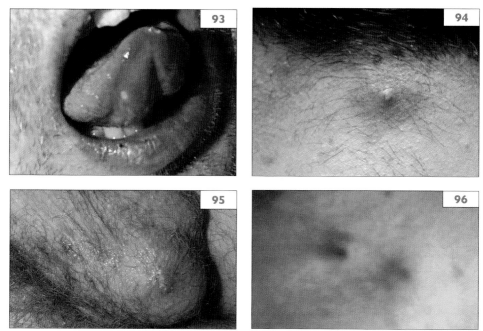

93–96 Mucocutaneous manifestations of Behçet's disease. 93: Painful oral apthous ulceration of the tongue; 94: papulopustular (acneiform) lesion (courtesy of Hasan Yazici, MD); 95: scrotal ulceration; 96: pathergy and venipuncture site.

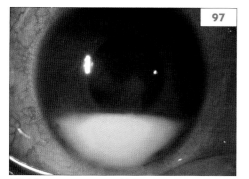

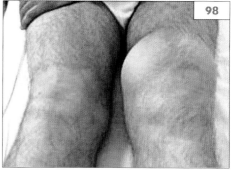

97 Hypopneon uveitis (debris in anterior chamber) in patient with Behçet's disease. (Courtesy of Hasan Yazici, MD.)

98 Nondeforming, nonerosive monoarticular arthritis in knee of patient with Behçet's disease. (Courtesy of Hasan Yazici, MD.)

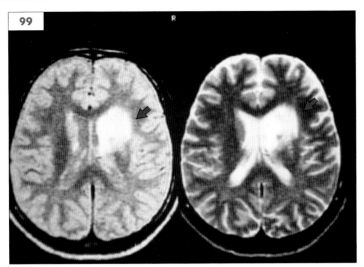

99 Parenchymal central nervous system involvement by MRI (arrows) in Behçet's disease. (Courtesy of Hasan Yazici, MD.)

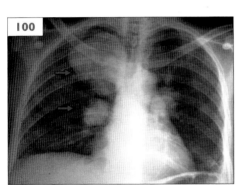

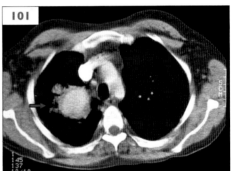

100, 101 Pulmonary artery aneurysm by chest radiograph (100, arrows) and CT (101, arrow) complicating Behçet's disease. (Courtesy of Hasan Yazici, MD.)

DIFFERENTIAL DIAGNOSIS

The most common considerations in the evaluation of BD include IBD, systemic lupus erythematosus (SLE), ReA, herpes simplex infection, recurrent aphthous stomatitis, and complex aphthosis.

Diagnostic criteria for BD are shown in *Table 27*.

INVESTIGATIONS

Laboratory findings are nonspecific. Anemia of chronic disease and leukocytosis are common. ESR and CRP are variably elevated and may be useful in tracking treatment response. IgA levels are commonly elevated. Other serologies including RF, ANA, and antineutrophil cytoplasmic antibody (ANCA) are typically negative. Complements are normal to high.

Imaging modalities may be helpful in select cases. With central nervous system (CNS) involvement in BD, MRI/CT may show parenchymal changes in the brain. Ventilation–perfusion (VQ) scans may reveal perfusion defects with pulmonary artery aneurysm. CT/CT angiogram may be needed to evaluate for pulmonary thrombosis, while lower extremity duplex scanning may be indicated with suspected deep venous thrombosis.

HISTOLOGY

Involved tissues show characteristic neutrophilic infiltrates and evidence of vasculitis.

PROGNOSIS

Overall mortality due to BD is low with most deaths occurring secondary to complications related to pulmonary artery aneurysms and CNS involvement. Ocular complications are a cause of significant morbidity.

MANAGEMENT

There is no standard management for BD. Current recommendations are based on small trials, case series, or historical use. Treatment selection is usually made on the basis of disease severity and organ system involvement, with the most aggressive treatment reserved for life-threatening disease:

- Mild mucocutaneous involvement: Topical or intralesional corticosteroids, colchicine or dapsone are the most often used for mild disease; penicillin has been shown in a few small studies to be of benefit.
- Severe mucocutaneous involvement: Thalidomide, MTX, oral corticosteroids, interferon-α, or TNF-α antagonists have all been advocated.
- Systemic disease: GCs, AZA, interferon (IFN)-α, CTX, and TNF-α antagonists have all been shown to be of benefit; embolization with immunosuppression (CTX) has been shown to be of most benefit to patients with pulmonary artery aneurysm.

Table 27 The International Study Group Diagnostic Criteria for Behçet's disease*

Recurrent oral ulceration (apthous or herpetiform) observed by the physician or patient recurring at least three times in one 12 month period

AND at least two of the following:

Recurrent genital ulceration

Eye lesions: anterior uveitis, posterior uveitis, cells in the vitreous by slit lamp examination, or retinal vasculitis observed by an ophthalmologist

Skin lesions: erythema nodosum, pseudofolliculitis, papulopustular lesions, or acneiform nodules in postadolescent patients not on corticosteroids

Pathergy read by a physician at 24–48 hours

* Assumes absence of other explantory conditions

Juvenile Idiopathic Arthritis

- Juvenile idiopathic arthritis
- Hereditary periodic fevers

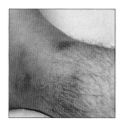 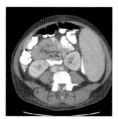 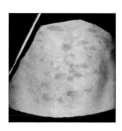 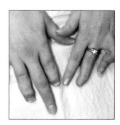

Juvenile idiopathic arthritis

DEFINITION

Juvenile idiopathic arthritis (JIA) is a term used to describe a group of chronic arthropathies involving individuals 16 years of age or younger. A diagnosis of JIA requires evidence of a persistent arthritis for at least 6 weeks. A subtype is delineated 6 months into the disease course based on number of joints involved and clinical characteristics (*Tables 28, 29*).

EPIDEMIOLOGY AND ETIOLOGY

The prevalence of JIA is estimated at 100–400 cases per 100 000 children. Yearly incidence in North America and Europe is estimated at 10–20 cases per 100 000 children. Oligoarticular JIA is the most common subtype (40% of cases) while polyarticular JIA is next most frequent (25%). Age of onset and gender varies by subtype with most cases presenting in girls between 1–3 years of age (for oligoarticular and seronegative polyarticular subtypes). Enthesitis-related arthritis (ERA) and juvenile psoriatic arthritis (PsA) present

---

Table 28 International League of Associations for Rheumatology (ILAR) definitions

Oligoarticular arthritis

Less than four joints in the first 6 months

If more than four joints become involved after 6 months, then the diagnoses becomes extended to oligoarticular JIA

Polyarticular arthritis

Five or more joints involved in the first 6 months of disease

Subdivided based on if a rheumatoid factor is positive on two occasions at least 3 months apart

Systemic arthritis

Arthritis in association with quotidian spiking fever of 2 weeks duration and one of the following:

Evanescent migratory rash

Hepatosplenomegaly

Serositis

Lymphadenopathy

Enthesitis-related arthritis

Arthritis and enthesitis (or)

Arthritis and/or enthesitis plus two of the following:

Sacroiliac joint or inflammatory back pain

HLA-B27 positivity

New onset arthritis in a male 6 years of age or older

First degree relative with history of HLA-B27-positive disease

Acute anterior uveitis

Psoriatic arthritis

Psoriasis and arthritis (or)

Arthritis plus two of the following:

Dactylitis

Nail changes (pitting or oncholysis)

Family history of psoriasis in a first-degree relative

Unclassified arthritis

Arthritis not fully fitting the above definitions or a mixture of two or more of the above

in late childhood and early adolescence. As children approach adulthood, the likelihood of rheumatoid factor (RF)-positive polyarthritis increases (*Table 30*). The etiology for most JIA subtypes remains largely unknown: however, there is strong evidence of both genetic and autoimmune influence.

Table 29 Clinical characteristics of JIA subtypes

Subtype	No. joints involved	Other characteristics
Oligoarticular arthritis	≤4 joints at 6 months	Chronic anterior uveitis; ANA positive 50–70%
Persistent	Remains ≤4 joints for duration of disease	
Extended	More than 4 joints become involved after first 6 months	
Polyarticular arthritis	≥5 joints at 6 months	
RF-negative	Asymmetric arthritis	Chronic anterior uveitis ANA + 20–40%
RF-positive	Symmetric arthritis	RF positive (×2); similar to adult RA
Systemic	Any number, symmetric	Fever, rash, LA, HSM, MAS
Enthesitis-related arthritis	Typically ≤4 joints, asymmetric	Male ≥6 yrs of age, HLA-B27+, AAU, axial involvement late (spine and SI joints)
Psoriatic arthritis	Typically ≤4 joints	Positive family history, dactylitis, nail changes

AAU: acute anterior uveitis; ANA: antinuclear antibody; HSM: hepatosplenomegaly; LA: lymphadenopathy; MAS: macrophage activation syndrome; RA: rheumatoid arthritis; RF: rheumatoid factor.

Table 30 Age of onset, gender distributions, and genetic associations based on juvenile idiopathic arthritis subtype

Subtype	Mean age of onset (years)	Female:male	Genetic HLA associations
Oligoarticular arthritis	1–3	4:1	DR8, DR5, A2
Polyarticular arthritis			
Rheumatoid factor negative	1–3	3:1	
Rheumatoid factor positive	9–12	9:1	DR4
Systemic	2–4	1:1	
Enthesitis-related arthritis	9–12	1:7	B27
Psoriatic arthritis	7–10	2:1	

PATHOGENESIS

T cells play an important role in the pathogenesis of oligo- and polyarticular JIA. Activated CD4+ T cell aggregates form early within the synovium. Chronic inflammation leads to destruction of cartilage and bone. The destruction is primarily a result of proinflammatory cytokines (tumor necrosis factor [TNF]-α, interleukin [IL]1, IL6, and so on) and metalloproteinase production from T cells and macrophages. Systemic arthritis may, in part, be driven by abnormal cytotoxic natural killer (NK) cell function which would help explain the increased risk of macrophage activation syndrome (MAS) in systemic JIA. The systemic manifestations of systemic JIA also appear to be primarily driven by IL-6 and less so IL-1. Similarities to pathogen-induced reactive arthritis (ReA) suggests that ERA may be associated with an infectious trigger in the context of HLA-B27. PsA seems to be mediated by activated CD8+ T cells which are found in higher numbers in both skin lesions and synovial fluid.

CLINICAL HISTORY AND PHYSICAL EXAMINATION
Oligoarticular JIA

- ≤4 joints involved in the first 6 months of disease; knee and/or ankle involvement at onset is common. Involvement of small joints, wrist, elbow, or temporomandibular joint (TMJ) is rare (involvement may predict extension to a polyarticular course).
- Systemic inflammation is uncommon.
- Primary extra-articular manifestation is chronic anterior iridocyclitis (uveitis), which affects ~20% of oligoarticular patients. There is an association with antinuclear antibody (ANA) positivity and is often asymptomatic, making regular ophthalmologic screening mandatory (*Table 31*).

RF-negative polyarticular JIA

- Upper extremity and small joint involvement is more common than in oligoarticular JIA; features are more asymmetric than in RF-positive JIA. TMJ involvement occurs and tenosynovitis is seen (in wrists, ankles, and flexor tendons of the hands).
- Chronic anterior uveitis is common (~10–15%) especially with ANA positivity (*Table 31*).

- Systemic inflammation can occur with low-grade fevers; rash, hepatosplenomegaly, lymphadenopathy, and serositis are rare.

RF-positive polyarticular JIA

- Symmetric arthritis of wrists and fingers is most common and tenosynovitis is common.
- Systemic inflammation is typical (elevations in erythrocyte sedimentation rate [ESR] and C-reactive protein [CRP]).
- Cervical spine (including atlanto–axial disease) and TMJ involvement are more common (**102**).
- Uveitis is rare; secondary Sjögren's syndrome may occur.
- Subcutaneous nodules are uncommon, but are strongly associated with subtype.

Systemic arthritis

- High spiking fever ≥39°C is found, in a quotidian pattern once or twice a day.
- Transient macular rash occurs at onset (~90%) most prominent during fevers, so can be described as transient.
- Arthritis can be delayed (weeks to even months) in some cases; abdominal or chest pain occurs secondary to pericarditis or pleuritis although serositis is often asymptomatic.
- Diffuse lymphadenopathy (~50%) and hepatosplenomegaly (~30–50%) (**103**) can occur.
- Arthritis is usually oligoarticular (polyarticular in ~25%) involving wrists, knees, and ankles.
- Uveitis is almost never observed.

ERA

Enthesitis is an early clinical feature (children/adolescents), associated with peripheral lower extremity arthritis. Involvement of insertion points of the Achilles tendon or plantar fascia is most common. Axial involvement can occur (e.g. sacroiliitis), but systemic manifestations are rare.

PsA

Arthritis is typically oligoarticular, of large and small joints. It can precede the rash by months to years. Dactylitis (~50%) and nail changes (nail pitting) are strongly associated with the subtype. Axial spine involvement occurs, as does chronic anterior uveitis, especially with ANA positivity (*Table 31*).

DIFFERENTIAL DIAGNOSIS

The differential diagnosis in JIA is broad and different for the different subtypes. Other entities that can mimic JIA include infection (particularly with systemic onset JIA), other connective tissue and autoimmune diseases (lupus, sarcoidosis, inflammatory bowel disease [IBD], ReA, vasculitis), inheritable diseases, malignancies including leukemia and neuroblastoma (particularly with oligoarticular disease), and trauma. MAS is a potentially life-threatening complication of JIA. Biologic agents used in the treatment of JIA include anti-TNF agents.

INVESTIGATIONS

- ESR and CRP: Significant elevations with a mono- or oligoarticular arthritis should raise concerns for infection, IBD, or malignancy; moderately elevated in polyarticular JIA; can track with treatment response; a falling ESR in patients with systemic arthritis who clinically appear to be worsening may indicate MAS secondary to fibrinogen consumption.
- Ferritin: often elevated in patients with systemic arthritis.

Table 31 Uveitis screening recommendations in juvenile idiopathic arthritis*

Subtype	ANA	Screening frequency (months) <7 years of age	Screening frequency (months) >7 years of age
Oligoarticular arthritis	+	3–4	6
	–	6	
RF-negative polyarticular	+	3–4	
	–	6	
RF-positive polyarticular	+/–	When symptomatic	When symptomatic
Systemic		12	12
Enthesitis-related		When symptomatic	When symptomatic
Psoriatic arthritis	+	3–4	6
	–	6	12

*If no uveitis is present after 4 years of disease activity, the screening level can decrease one level.

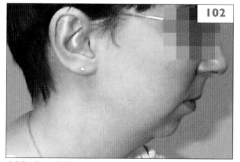

102 An adult patient who had been diagnosed with rheumatoid factor-positive polyarticular juvenile idiopathic arthritis; marked temporomandibular involvement resulting in micrognathia. (Courtesy of Dr GF Moore.)

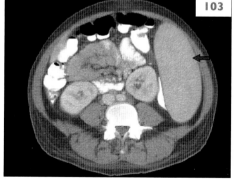

103 CT of abdomen in a patient with systemic juvenile idiopathic arthritis showing marked splenomegaly (arrow). (Courtesy of Dr GF Moore.)

- Complete blood count (CBC): Evaluation for a malignancy or viral process; leukocytosis is seen with systemic arthritis; anemia of chronic disease (polyarticular and systemic JIA).
- Lactate dehydrogenase (LDH)/uric acid: Evaluation for underlying leukemia (particularly with nocturnal pain).
- RF: Rarely useful as a screening test (5–10% positivity in JIA *vs.* 1–4% in healthy children); RF positivity with polyarthritis is suggestive of a more aggressive clinical course.
- ANA: Not useful as a screening test for JIA; ANA is associated with a higher uveitis risk once JIA is established.

- Imaging: Periarticular erosions (particularly in RF-positive polyarthritis) and juxta-articular osteoporosis are common (**104, 105**); cervical spine imaging should be done in all patients prior to clearing for contact sports.
- Synovial fluid analysis: Inflammatory fluid with polymorphonuclear leukocyte (PMN) predominance is important in excluding infection.

PROGNOSIS

Most (40–60%) of JIA patients achieve inactive disease with long-term follow-up. A majority of patients regardless of subtype require persistent medications to achieve a lasting clinical remission. Poor prognostic indicators include a symmetric polyarthritis, early wrist or hip involvement, RF positivity, or early radiographic changes. Oligoarthritis patients generally have the best prognosis with 25–50% achieving remission 6–10 years after disease onset. RF-positive polyarthritis patients follow a course similar to adults with a progressive and often deforming arthritis. Systemic

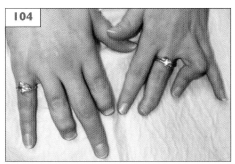

104 Hands of adult patient diagnosed during childhood with rheumatoid factor-positive juvenile idiopathic arthritis; note marked bone length discrepancies (e.g. second and fourth digits of right hand) and deformity.

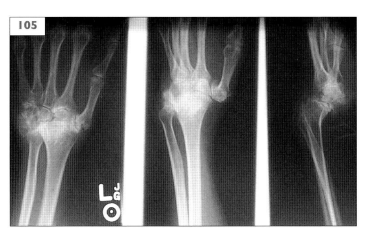

105 Hand radiographs in a patient with juvenile idiopathic arthritis showing marked destructive changes involving wrists.

arthritis follows three patterns where half of patients experience a monocyclic or intermittent course with periods of remission and relatively easily-controlled disease exacerbation. The other 50% suffer a chronic unremitting course typically characterized by a persistent arthritis with minimal systemic features. Approximately 40% of PsA patients will have chronic, active disease.

MANAGEMENT

JIA management is dictated by the severity of subtype of disease, incorporating both pharmacological and nonpharmacological approaches. Medications commonly used in the treatment of JIA include nonsteroidal anti-inflammatory drugs (NSAIDs), corticosteroids (particularly intra-articular), biologic and nonbiologic disease-modifying antirheumatic drugs (DMARDs). Methotrexate (MTX; 0.3–1 mg/kg weekly up to a maximum of 25 mg per week) is the most commonly used nonbiologic DMARD. IL-1 inhibition (e.g. anakinra) may play a special role in the treatment of systemic JIA.

Hereditary periodic fevers

DEFINITION

The hereditary periodic fevers are a collection of rare disorders characterized by high fevers, serosal inflammation, arthralgias/arthritis, and cutaneous manifestations. Inborn errors of the innate immune system result in inflammation, and many experts thus refer to these diseases as 'autoinflammatory diseases'. This group of disorders is often classified by the mechanism of inheritance (*Table 32*).

EPIDEMIOLOGY AND ETIOLOGY

With the advent of the Human Genome Project, the precise genetic defects leading to disease conditions have been identified:

- The *MEFV* (MEditerranean FeVer) gene on chromosome 16 contains the missense mutation found in most cases of familial Mediterranean fever (FMF). This genetic mutation is not uncommon in Mediterranean populations, including Sephardic Jews, Armenians, Turks, Arabs, and Greeks. However, FMF remains rare (though the most prevalent of this collection of diseases), with perhaps 10 000 cases worldwide, indicating that penetrance is incomplete.

Table 32 Inheritance patterns in hereditary periodic fevers

Disorder	Inheritance
Familial Mediterranean fever (FMF)	Autosomal recessive
Hypergammaglobulinemia D with periodic fever syndrome (HIDS)	Autosomal recessive
Tumor necrosis factor receptor superfamily 1A-associated periodic syndrome (TRAPS)	Autosomal dominant
Familial cold autoinflammatory syndrome (FCAS)	Autosomal dominant
Muckle–Wells	Autosomal dominant
Neonatal-onset multisystem inflammatory disease (NOMID)	Autosomal dominant

- TNF receptor superfamily 1A-associated periodic syndrome (TRAPS) was formerly known as familial Hibernian fever, reflecting its manifestation in northern European populations. As its worldwide distribution seems to be greater than originally appreciated, it has been renamed to reflect the gene associated with the disease.
- Hypergammaglobulinemia D with periodic fever syndrome (HIDS), like FMF, is recessively inherited, and the gene responsible is the *MVK* (mevalonate kinase) gene on chromosome 12. This rare disease is predominately of the Dutch and French, but is found globally.
- Familial cold autoinflammatory syndrome (FCAS), Muckle–Wells syndrome, and neonatal-onset multisystem inflammatory disease (NOMID) represent a continuum of diseases associated with varying defects in the cold-induced, autoinflammatory syndrome-1 (*CIAS1*) gene. This gene encodes a protein named cryopyrin (described later), and thus these diseases are collectively known as the 'cryopyrinopathies'.

PATHOGENESIS
The pathogenesis of each of these disorders is unique, though all are caused by inherited genetic mutations. These mutations lead to dysfunction of the innate immune system leading to systemic inflammation. As noted above, FMF results from mutations in the *MEFV* gene. This gene encodes for the protein pyrin, which is expressed in leukocytes and fibroblasts. Pyrin is involved with the inhibition of various cytokines, including the inflammatory mediator IL-1β. Simplified, the defected *MEFV* gene leads to loss of inhibition of inflammation in FMF. Similarly, a genetic defect in TRAPS is responsible for inflammation, though in this disorder a gain of function mutation is observed in the *TNFRSF1A* gene. The exact pathogenesis remains uncertain. Patients with HIDS have a defect in the aforementioned *MVK* gene which encodes for mevalonate kinase. Complete inhibition of this enzyme results in the severe phenotype known as mevalonic aciduria, while HIDS patients have only a partial reduction in the activity of mevalonate kinase. This enzyme is involved in production of cholesterols, leading some to experiment with

upstream inhibition of HMG-CoA reductase inhibitors ('statins') as treatment. Lastly, the cryopyrinopathies all result from various mutations in the *CIAS1* gene. This gene encodes for cryopyrin, a protein that combines with other proteins to form an inflammasome. The inflammasome activates caspase-1, which in turn cleaves procytokines (such as pro-IL-1β) into the active forms. The exact mechanism resulting from this genetic defect remains elusive.

CLINICAL HISTORY AND PHYSICAL EXAMINATION
Exacerbations of disease manifest with fevers, often with shaking chills. The duration of exacerbations varies; whereas FMF attacks last less than 4 days, TRAPS attacks can infrequently last for weeks. Despite the term 'periodic', there is usually no pattern to the frequency of attacks, and even the length of attacks can vary in an individual patient. Stress, infections, trauma, and even menses have been associated with triggering of attacks. In addition to fever, serositis is a common finding, usually manifested by abdominal pain, but also pleuritis, pericarditis, and even scrotitis (the tunica vaginalis is a remnant of the peritoneal membrane). Articular manifestations are also common during attacks, ranging from arthralgias to overt arthritis. Cutaneous disorders range from the erysipelas-like erythema in FMF (**106**) to the urticarias associated with the cryopyrinopathies (**107**). With longer disease duration, amyloidosis (AA type) is the most feared complication (**108, 109**). Small subsets of patients demonstrate the unfortunate signs and symptoms of end-organ failure (usually renal) as the initial clinical presentation. In addition to ethnicity, certain physical signs and symptoms can help differentiate these disorders (*Table 33*).

DIFFERENTIAL DIAGNOSIS
The differential diagnosis evolves with duration of symptoms. Early in the course of disease, infections and neoplasms may be suspected based on signs and symptoms. However, as the duration of disease lengthens, occult infections or malignancies become less likely. At this stage, other autoimmune disorders are commonly entertained, including JIA, adult-onset Still's disease, IBD, sarcoidosis, and Behçet's disease (BD).

The diagnosis of the hereditary periodic fever syndromes is made clinically, but is often augmented by genetic testing.

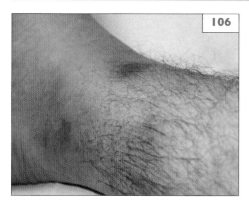

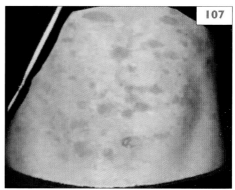

106 Erythematous erysipelas-like rash occurring on the ankle of a patient with familial Mediterranean fever (FMF) during an acute attack. (With permission, BioMed Central, London; Lachmann & Hawkins, *Arthritis Res Therapy* 2009; **11**:210.)

107 Rash occurring in a young patient with Muckle–Wells syndrome; the rash resolved after therapy with IL-1 receptor antagonist. (With permission, John Wiley, NJ; Hawkins, *et al.*, *Arthritis Rheum* 2004; **50**:607–12.)

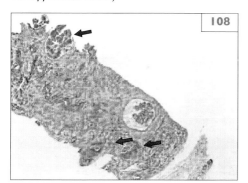

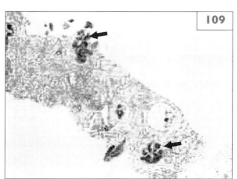

108, 109 Renal biopsy specimen from a patient with long-standing hypergammaglobulinemia D with periodic fever syndrome (HIDS) complicated by amyloidosis. Amorphous amyloid deposits in glomeruli with positive Congo red staining (**108**, arrows) and positive immunohistochemistry with antiserum amyloid monoclonal antibody (**109**, arrows). (With permission, John Wiley, NJ; Lachmann, *et al.*, *Arthritis Rheum* 2006; **54**:2010–4.)

Table 33 Clinical features unique to the different types of hereditary periodic fevers

Disorder	Unique clinical feature
Hypergammaglobulinemia D with periodic fever syndrome (HIDS)	Lymphadenopathy during attacks
Tumor necrosis factor receptor superfamily 1A-associated periodic syndrome (TRAPS)	Ocular findings including conjunctivitis and periorbital edema
Muckle–Wells syndrome	Sensorineural hearing loss
Neonatal-onset multisystem inflammatory disease (NOMID)	Constant, daily rash

INVESTIGATIONS

Laboratory findings (aside from previously discussed genetic testing) are relatively nonspecific in this class of disorders. Acute phase reactants such as the ESR and CRP are elevated during attacks, and often between acute attacks as well. Leukocytosis is also common during attacks, as is hypergammaglobulinemia (often IgD). Many of these disorders share the long-term complication of amyloidosis, such that serum amyloid A levels are frequently elevated. Imaging tests (including chest radiograph, abdominal ultrasound, and/or computed tomography [CT], and echocardiography) may be necessary in the evaluation of serositis.

PROGNOSIS

Permanent end-organ damage and death remain rare outcomes, and when they occur, are often due to a common complication of these disorders, amyloidosis (**108, 109**).

MANAGEMENT

Treatment varies for each of the specific disorders:

- FMF is unique in its dramatic response to oral colchicine, both in resolution of acute attacks and prevention of attacks and amyloidosis. Due to toxicity, there is no role for intravenous colchicine.
- TRAPS is initially responsive to corticosteroids, but this response diminishes over time. Unfortunately, colchicine is ineffective in TRAPS. Etanercept (a biologic agent targeting TNF) has been effective in TRAPS.
- HIDS generally responds poorly to both colchicine and corticosteroids.

Traditional steroid-sparing agents such as MTX and azathioprine (AZA) are most often ineffective among these diseases. IL-1 receptor antagonist anakinra has received favorable reports in many of these diseases including the cryopyrinopathies. Aside from managing pharmacotherapy, the most important role of the physician is continued surveillance for complications of disease. Early detection of amyloidosis is important, even if management remains difficult. As the kidney is the organ most often affected by amyloidosis in these diseases, routine urinalyses should be performed screening for proteinuria.

Connective Tissue Diseases

- Raynaud's phenomenon
- Sjögren's syndrome
- Systemic lupus erythematosus
- Drug-induced lupus
- Antiphospholipid antibody syndrome
- Polymyositis and dermatomyositis
- Systemic sclerosis (scleroderma)
- Mixed connective tissue disease and undifferentiated connective tissue disease
- Relapsing polychondritis

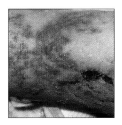 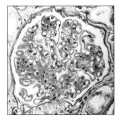 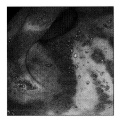 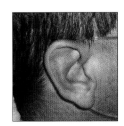

Raynaud's phenomenon

DEFINITION

Raynaud's' phenomenon (RP) is an exaggerated response to cold temperature or emotional stress that results in transient digital ischemia. RP is considered primary if these symptoms occur alone without evidence of any associated rheumatic disorders. RP is considered secondary when it occurs as a manifestation of another health condition or exposure. Rheumatic conditions associated with secondary RP include scleroderma (SSc) (where RP is nearly universal), lupus, Sjögren's syndrome, dermatomyositis, mixed connective tissue disease (MCTD), and rheumatoid arthritis (RA).

EPIDEMIOLOGY AND ETIOLOGY

The prevalence of RP ranges between 4% and 16% in women and between 3% and 6% in men. The frequency and severity of the 'attacks' are influenced by the daily ambient temperature, with exacerbations during cold weather. Primary RP is much more common than secondary RP. The prevalence of secondary RP in SSc is greater than 95%, whereas in most other connective tissue disorders (CTDs) it is approximately 20–30%. The median age at the onset of primary RP is 14 years with around one-quarter of patients experiencing onset at the age of 40 years of age and older.

PATHOGENESIS

The signs and symptoms of RP are due to vasoconstriction of the digital arteries, precapillary arterioles, and cutaneous arteriovenous shunts. RP pathogenesis may be explained on the basis of dysregulated neuroendothelial control mechanisms. The key issue is the imbalance between vasoconstriction and vasodilation (in favor of vasoconstriction). Evidence points to abnormalities in the blood vessel wall (endothelium and smooth muscle), in the neural control of the vascular tone, and in circulating mediators (including those produced as a result of platelet activation and of oxidative stress).

CLINICAL HISTORY AND PHYSICAL EXAMINATION

RP most often affects the hands, but may also affect the toes and occasionally areas of the face. 'Attacks' may be precipitated by fluctuations in ambient temperature, exercise, emotional stress, or other triggers. These attacks are typically transient, lasting 15–20 minutes but may vary in duration, frequency, and severity.

RP is classically characterized by the sudden development of cold/painful digits with classic triphasic skin color changes: Pallor (white) with initial ischemia → cyanosis (blue) with deoxygenation → reperfusion (red), usually with rewarming.

A Raynaud's attack typically begins in a single finger and then spreads to other digits symmetrically in both hands. The index, middle, and 'ring' finger are the most frequently involved digits, while the thumb is often spared (**110**). RP may be associated with sensations of 'pins and needles,' numbness, and finger ache. In severe secondary RP, pain or ulceration of the skin may result from critical ischemia. In SSc, RP is often the presenting feature and it can be a major cause of morbidity.

A complete physical examination is mandatory to evaluate for signs of rheumatic conditions associated with secondary RP (*Table 34*). An abnormal nailfold capillary examination (the presence of dilated capillary loops and 'drop-outs') may be indicative of secondary RP.

DIFFERENTIAL DIAGNOSIS

The diagnosis of RP is clinical. Reports of exaggerated sensitivity to cold temperatures are common among the general population. Cool skin and nondemarcated mottling of the skin of the digits (e.g. acrocyanosis), hands, and limbs are considered a normal response to the cold exposure. Distinguishing primary from secondary RP is critical; the latter is more commonly associated with severe attacks and the development of digital ulcerations.

Most patients with RP report symmetric involvement of the digits. With asymmetric involvement, a mechanical occlusion of the large vessel should be considered. An occupational history of 'vibratory tool' use may suggest secondary RP due to 'hand–arm vibration syndrome'. With digital ischemia, particularly in the absence of 'classic' RP, an evaluation for alternative etiologies including thromboembolic disease and systemic vasculitis may be warranted.

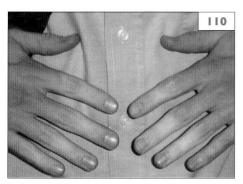

110

110 Patient with primary Raynaud's phenomenon; note the demarcation of skin color changes and symmetric involvement of multiple digits. (Courtesy of Dr GF Moore.)

Table 34 Conditions associated with secondary Raynaud's phenomenon

Rheumatic disease
Scleroderma
Systemic lupus erythematosus
Mixed connective tissue disease
Dermatomyositis/polymyositis
Sjögren's syndrome
Undifferentiated connective tissue disorder
Rheumatoid arthritis
Antiphospholipid antibody syndrome

Hematologic disorders
Cryoglobulinemia
Polycythemia vera
Cold agglutinin disease
Cryofibrinogenemia
Waldendstrom's macroglobulinemia

Endocrine disorders
Hypothyroidism
Carcinoid syndrome
Pheochromocytoma

Environmental agents and injury
Frostbite
Repetitive occupational stress (hand–arm vibration syndrome)
Hypothenar hammer syndrome
Vasospasm
Migraine headaches

Vascular embolus or occlusion
Cardiac thrombus

Neuropathy
Carpal tunnel syndrome
Thoracic outlet syndrome

Drugs and toxins
Chemotherapeutic agents (bleomycin, cisplatin, carboplatin, vinblastine)
Sympathomimetic drugs (decongestants, diet pills, amphetamines)
Serotonin agonists (sumatriptan)
Ergotamines
Estrogen
Nicotine
Narcotics
Cyclosporine
Clonidine
Cocaine
Polyvinyl chloride
Nonselective beta blockers

Diagnostic criteria

A diagnosis of RP may be made if the patient provides a history of cold sensitivity and a history of the classic triad of sequential digital pallor, cyanosis, and rubor following cold exposure. Screening questions to ask are:

1 Are your fingers unusually sensitive to cold?
2 Do your fingers change color when they are exposed to cold temperatures?
3 Do they turn white, blue, or both?

The diagnosis of RP is confirmed by a positive response to all three questions. The diagnosis is excluded if the responses to questions two and three are negative. Several clinical characteristics may help to distinguish patients with primary from those with secondary RP (*Table 35*).

INVESTIGATIONS

If after a complete history and a physical examination (including capillary nailfold microscopy), there is a low suspicion of an underlying disease, then there is no need for further specialized tests and a diagnosis of primary RP is established. Select laboratory and/or imaging studies are used when secondary RP is suspected:

- Complete blood count (CBC), electrolytes, glucose, creatinine, liver function tests, thyroid stimulating hormone, urinalysis, erythrocyte sedimentation rate (ESR), antinuclear antibody (ANA), rheumatoid factor (RF), serum protein and immunoelectrophoresis, cryoglobulins.
- In ANA-positive patients, tests for the anticentromere and antitopoisomerase (anti-Scl-70) antibodies are indicated.
- Electromyography (EMG) or nerve conduction studies should be performed when nerve compression is a possibility.
- Vascular Doppler studies may help in the assessment of the several forms of secondary RP.
- A chest and/or cervical radiograph may help to reveal a bony cervical rib in the case of thoracic obstruction syndrome.

PROGNOSIS

Primary RP has an excellent prognosis while 5–10% of patients will evolve into an autoimmune condition. The prognosis of secondary RP is dependent on the underlying condition and is more commonly associated with painful episodes, the development of ischemic digital ulcerations, and tissue loss (**111**).

Table 35 Clinical characteristics helpful in distinguishing primary from secondary Raynaud's phenomenon (RP)

Primary RP	Secondary RP
Female	Age of onset >30 years
Onset often in teens or 20s	Pain associated with episodes
Vasospastic attacks precipitated by cold or emotional stress	Asymmetric attacks
Symmetric attacks involving both hands	Signs of tissue ischemia
Absence of tissue necrosis, gangrene, or digital pitting	Signs or symptoms suggestive of a connective tissue disorder (arthritis, myalgias, fever, dry mucous membranes, rashes, abnormal lung function)
No history or physical findings suggestive of a secondary cause	Abnormal nailfold capillaries
Normal nailfold capillaries	Presence of antibodies against a specific autoantigen (anticentromere or anti-Scl-70)
Normal erythrocyte sedimentation rate	
Negative serological findings	
Symptoms present for >2 years without the appearance of an underlying cause	

MANAGEMENT

Avoidance of known triggers including cold exposures are critical; education on the importance of maintaining core body temperature (layering) is important. Avoidance of smoking/passive smoking is prudent. Sympathomimetic drugs should be avoided.

Medications are indicated for moderate to severe primary or secondary RP:

- Vasodilators – first line. Calcium channels blockers (dihydropyridines: nifedepine, amlodipine) are often first line; slow release preparations are preferred.
- Aspirin (81 mg) is recommended in select patients with severe RP, those at risk for digital ulceration, or larger artery thrombotic events.
- Angiotensin-converting enzyme (ACE) inhibitors/angiotensin receptor blockers (ARBs) may improve digital blood flow; losartan has been shown to decrease the number/severity of attacks.
- Sympatholytic agents (prazosin, an α-1 receptor blocker) may be beneficial, but clinical improvement may not be sustained.
- Topical nitrates may reduce the number/ severity of attacks.
- Prostaglandins: Iloprost is used to treat severe pulmonary hypertension and critical ischemia in patients with RP.
- Endothelin receptor antagonist (bosentan) is used in the treatment of severe pulmonary hypertension and for prevention of digital ulcers in patients with SSc.
- Phosphodiesterase inhibitors (sildenafil, tadalafil) may reduce the severity of RP attacks.
- Selective serotonin reuptake inhibitors (fluoxetine) have limited data, but may improve RP symptoms.
- Statins have a vasculoprotective effect.
- Sympathectomy is used to ligate the sympathetic nerves that cause vasoconstriction; localized digital sympathectomy is preferred.

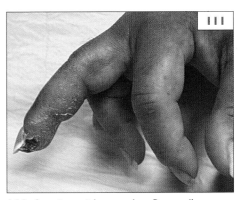

111 A patient with secondary Raynaud's phenomenon (with a history of scleroderma) presenting with a digital ulceration and subsequent loss of digital pulp. (Courtesy of Dr GF Moore.)

Sjögren's syndrome

DEFINITION
Sjögren's syndrome (SS) is a slowly progressive autoimmune disease that exhibits a wide range of manifestations, most commonly associated with exocrine gland dysfunction (e.g. salivary and lacrimal glands) due to lymphocytic infiltration.

EPIDEMIOLOGY AND ETIOLOGY
SS is a relatively common autoimmune disorder and prevalence estimates range from 0.5% to 5%. Approximately one-half of all cases are primary SS with the remaining secondary (occurring in association with other autoimmune diseases including RA, lupus, and SSc among others). Primary SS is much more common in women than men with a bimodal age of onset: the first during the third to fourth decades of life and the second following menopause in women. Although the majority of cases occur in midlife, the disorder can be seen in children and the elderly.

The etiology of SS is not well understood, although there has been substantial speculation that persistent viral infections may play an important role in 'triggering' SS in genetically susceptible individuals.

PATHOGENESIS
The glandular epithelial cells play a critical role in contributing to the pathogenesis of SS. The glandular epithelial cells found in patients who have SS are immunologically activated, expressing major histocompatibility (MHC) class I and II molecules and B7 co-stimulatory molecules. These epithelial cells also produce proinflammatory cytokines and chemokines that attract lymphocytes, producing the characteristic periductal focal lymphocytic infiltrate with T-helper cells, B cells, and plasma cells.

CLINICAL HISTORY AND PHYSICAL EXAMINATION
Many symptoms of SS are nonspecific and the spectrum of clinical manifestations is broad. Because SS is frequently seen in middle-aged women, symptoms of cutaneous, oral, and vaginal dryness may initially be attributed to menopause. Symptoms of dry mouth are common to many conditions and are subjective. In SS, ~ 67% of patients report dry eyes and 93% report dry mouth. The clinical manifestations of SS may be categorized based on an exocrine gland or 'extraglandular' origin.

Exocrine gland features
- Ocular manifestations: Xerophthalmia (dry eyes) is the most prominent ocular manifestation; symptoms include foreign body-type sensation, inability to tolerate contact lenses, photosensitivity, eye fatigue, erythema, decreased visual acuity, discharge/'matting.'
- Oral manifestations: Xerostomia; inability to chew and swallow certain foods, such as a biscuit cracker, without drinking fluids (so-called 'cracker sign'); dysgusia; increased frequency of dental caries; oral thrush (fungal infection can present with oral sensitivity, erythema and loss of filiform papillae); angular cheilitis; swelling of parotid, sublingual, and/or submandibular glands (superimposed sialadenitis, usually, staphylococcal or pneumococcal can occur) (**112**).
- Other xeroses: Diminished glandular secretions can lead to dryness of the nose, throat, and trachea that results in hoarseness and chronic nonproductive cough. Involvement of the exocrine glands of the skin leads to skin dryness. Vaginal dryness may lead to pruritis, irritation, and dyspareunia.

Extraglandular features
- Systemic/vascular manifestations: RP; palpable and nonpalpable purpura in association with cryoglobulinemia and hyperglobulinemia (small-vessel vasculitis, **113**); urticarial vasculitis; necrotizing vasculitis of medium-sized vessels, as well as venous and arterial thrombosis.
- Musculoskeletal: Myalgias/arthralgias are common, nonerosive arthritis, myositis.
- Pulmonary: Obstructive airway disease, pulmonary infiltrates (pseudolymphoma or lymphocytic interstitial pneumonitis), fibrosing alveolitis.
- Renal (approximately one-third): Tubulointerstitial nephritis (TIN) with renal tubular acidosis type I, chronic interstitial nephritis, glomerulonephritis (uncommon).
- Gastrointestinal (GI)/hepatic: Esophageal stenosis, atrophic gastritis, pancreatitis,

primary biliary cirrhosis, chronic active hepatitis, cryptogenic cirrhosis.
- Neurological manifestations (~20%): Central nervous system (CNS) involvement, cranial neuropathies, myelopathy, and peripheral neuropathies.
- Autoimmune thyroid disease (frequently seen concomitantly with SS).

- Malignancy: Risk of non-Hodgkin's lymphoma is substantially increased (**114**); risk factors include parotid gland enlargement, splenomegaly, lymphadenopathy, palpable purpura, leg ulcers, hypocomplementemia, type II cryoglobulinemia, and cross-reactive idiotypes of monoclonal RF.

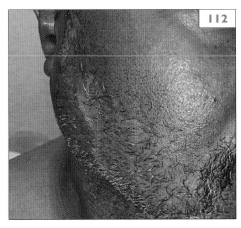

112 Patient with Sjögren's syndrome, xerostomia, and marked swelling of the parotid glands. (Courtesy of Dr GF Moore.)

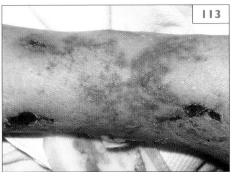

113 Purpura in Sjögren's syndrome patients may occur in association with cryoglobulinemia and hyperglobulinemia. (Courtesy of Dr GF Moore.)

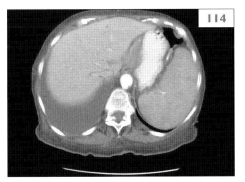

114 CT scan of the abdomen in a patient with Sjögren's syndrome complicated by lymphoma, demonstrating marked splenomegaly. (Courtesy of Dr GF Moore.)

DIFFERENTIAL DIAGNOSIS

The differential diagnosis for SS is summarized in *Table 36*. Diagnostic criteria for SS are shown in *Table 37*.

INVESTIGATIONS

- Schirmer tear test: Measures tear formation via placement of filter paper in the lower conjunctival sac; if <5 mm of paper is wet after 5 minutes, the test result is positive (**115**).
- Rose Bengal staining may be helpful to detect damaged conjunctival epithelium.
- Sialometry measures unstimulated salivary flow into a calibrated tube for 15 minutes.
- Parotid gland sialography is performed by introducing dye into the parotid duct.
- Minor salivary biopsy is highly specific; it typically involves a biopsy of the lip. Focal lymphocytic sialadenitis is defined as multiple, dense aggregates of 50 or more lymphocytes (1 focus) in perivascular or periductal areas in the majority of sampled glands (a characteristic histopathologic feature of SS).
- Serological and laboratory:
  - Diffuse hypergammaglobulinemia – 80%
  - Elevated ESR – 80%
  - Positive RF – 50–80%
  - Positive ANA – 70%
  - Circulating cryoglobulins –30%
  - Anemia – 40%
  - Leukopenia <30%
  - Antibodies to soluble acidic nuclear antigens (Ro/SSA and La/SSB). Anti-Ro/SSA observed in ~70% of patients with primary SS.

HISTOLOGY

The histological hallmark is a focal lymphocytic infiltration of the affected glands. B cell activation is a consistent finding in patients with SS and B and T cells invade and destroy target organs. Focal lymphocytic sialadenitis, defined as multiple, dense aggregates of 50 or more lymphocytes (1 focus) in perivascular or periductal areas in the majority of sampled glands, is a characteristic histopathologic feature of SS.

PROGNOSIS

SS is characterized by chronic courses and variable progression. The overall mortality is not increased compared with that of the general population. In subgroups of SS patients who have previously described risk factors for developing lymphoma, there is higher mortality.

MANAGEMENT

Therapy for SS is based on three major components:

- Moisture replacement:
  - Artificial tears: solutions consisting of methylcellulose/polyvinyl alcohol; dosage varies widely.
  - Temporary occlusion of the puncta through insertion of the plugs (collagen or silicone) or permanent occlusion by electrocautery can be used.
  - Sugarless gum/drops may help stimulate salivary flow.
- Stimulation of endogenous secretion:
  - Pilocarpine is a cholinergic/parasympathetic agent; it is indicated for xerostomia secondary to salivary gland hypofunction and contraindicated in patients with asthma, iritis, and narrow-angle glaucoma.
  - Cevimeline is a cholinergic agent that binds to muscarinic receptors and increases secretions of exocrine glands; side-effects include sweating, nausea, exacerbation of asthma, and cardiac abnormalities.
- Systemic/immnomodulatory treatment:
  - Nonsteroidal anti-inflammatory drugs (NSAIDs) for minor musculoskeletal symptoms of SS.
  - Hydroxychloroquine (HCQ) may improve features of immunologic reactivity; it is used for the treatment of arthralgias, myalgias, and constitutional symptoms.
  - Corticosteroid use is generally limited to the treatment of severe extraglandular manifestations of SS.
  - Patients with SS should undergo regular dental and ophthalmological evaluation as part of their care.

Table 36 Differential diagnosis of Sjögren's syndrome

Infection
Viral: Coxsackie virus, mumps, cytomegalovirus, human immunodeficiency virus, hepatitis
Bacterial: Acute sialadenitis (e.g. *Staphylococcus* or *Streptococcus* infection)
Fungal: Actinomycosis or histoplasmosis

Granulomatous disease
Sarcoidosis

Systemic diseases
Cirrhosis, diabetes mellitus, hyperlipoproteinemia, obesity, pregnancy and lactation, Cushing's disease, cystic fibrosis

Nutritional deficiency
Starvation, vitamin deficiency (B6, C, A)

Other infiltrative disorders
Malignancy of the parotid gland, leukemia, amyloidosis, lymphoma, pseudolyphoma

Drugs (associated with xerostomia)
Sedatives, hypnotics, narcotics, phenothiazine, atropine, propantheline, antiparkinsonian drugs, antihistamines, ephedrine, epinephrine, amphetamine

Table 37 Diagnostic criteria for Sjögren's syndrome (SS); American–European classification criteria (95% sensitivity and 95% specificity)*

Criteria
Symptoms of dry eye
Signs of dry eye (abnormal result of Schirmer or Rose Bengal test)
Symptoms of dry mouth
Minor salivary gland (lip) biopsy (focus score >1)
Tests indicating impaired salivary gland function (abnormal flow rate, scintigram, or sialogram)
Presence of autoantibodies (anti-Ro/SSA and/or anti-La/SSB)

Exclusion criteria
Past head and neck radiation treatment
Hepatitis C infection
Acquired immunodeficiency syndrome
Pre-existing lymphoma
Sarcoidosis
Graft versus host disease
Use of anticholinergic drugs

* To establish diagnosis of SS, four criteria must be present, with one of the four being objective measurement (biopsy or antibodies); exclusion criteria should be absent.

115 Schirmer test (used to detect deficient tear production) is performed by placing a filter paper strip at the junction of the eyelid margins; after 5 minutes, 15 mm of paper should be moistened if tear production is normal. Patients with Sjögren's syndrome have less moistening. (Courtesy of Dr GF Moore.)

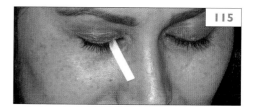

Systemic lupus erythematosus

DEFINITION
Systemic lupus erythematosus (SLE) is a multisystem, autoimmune disease that is heterogeneous in its presentation and manifestations; it is almost universally characterized by the presence of circulating ANA.

EPIDEMIOLOGY AND ETIOLOGY
SLE primarily affects young women with a peak incidence between the ages of 15 and 40 years, with a female to male ratio of 6 to 10:1. In the very young and the older patients, the female to male ratio is closer to 2:1. In the general population, SLE affects approximately one in 2000 individuals.

Though most cases of SLE appear sporadically, as is seen in other autoimmune conditions, there are genetic (heritable complement deficiency, HLA alleles, and PTPN22) and environmental (infection, sex hormones) factors that impact disease expression. There is a higher incidence of disease among first-degree relatives, and in monozygotic twins disease concordance is 25–50%. Of note, first-degree relatives of patients with SLE also appear to be at a higher risk for developing other autoimmune diseases including idiopathic thrombocytopenic purpura and autoimmune thyroiditis, suggesting shared genetic and/or environmental risk factors among these different conditions.

PATHOGENESIS
SLE is characterized by a loss of tolerance to self antigen and the expression of autoantibody (classically ANA). Inflammatory lesions in SLE are due to autoantibody binding to self antigen, the formation and deposition of immune complexes, complement activation, and the expression of proinflammatory cytokines (typically Th-2 phenotype, interleukin [IL]-4, IL-10).

CLINICAL HISTORY AND PHYSICAL EXAMINATION
SLE is manifested by a protean of different signs and symptoms leading to substantial clinical heterogeneity. Virtually every organ system can be affected in SLE, evident in the American College of Rheumatology (ACR) disease classification criteria (*Table 38*). Clinical signs and symptoms by system are summarized in *Table 39*.

DIFFERENTIAL DIAGNOSIS
The differential diagnosis for SLE is broad and is guided by the organ involvement and clinical presentation. In the hospitalized, acutely ill patient, infection and malignancy must be considered. Additionally, vasculitis and other CTDs can be confused with SLE. The key to a successful diagnosis is a complete history and physical examination coupled with appropriately targeted laboratory testing. Inflammatory arthritis of SLE may closely resemble that of RA,

---

Table 38 Revised American College of Rheumatology systemic lupus erythematosus classification criteria*

Malar rash

Discoid rash

Photosensitivity

Oral ulcers

Arthritis which is nonerosive involving two or more peripheral joints

Serositis to include pleuritis or pericarditis

Renal disorder to include persistent proteinuria (>500 mg per day or >3+ if quantification is not completed) or cellular casts (red cell, hemoglobin, granular, tubular, or mixed)

Neurological disorders to include seizures or psychosis

Hematological disorders to include hemolytic anemia, or leukopenia (<4000/mm³ total), or lymphopenia (<1500/mm³ on two or more occasions), or thrombocytopenia (<100 000/mm³ in the absence of offending drugs)

Immunological disorders to include anti-dsDNA antibody, or anti-Smith antibody, or positive findings of antiphospholipid antibodies (based on an abnormal serum level of IgG or IgM anticardiolipin antibodies or a positive lupus anticoagulant, or a false-positive serological test for syphilis)

ANA positivity by immunofluorescence or equivalent assay at any point in time, in the absence of drugs known to be associated with drug-induced lupus

* SLE diagnosis requires the presence of at least four criteria; criteria intended to ensure uniform patient populations in clinical trials; criteria need not be seen simultaneously and are often observed additively. ANA: antinuclear antibody; dsDNA: double stranded deoxyribonucleic acid; Ig: immunoglobulin.

Table 39 Clinical signs and symptoms in systemic lupus erythematosus

System	Signs/symptoms	Comments
Constitutional	Fevers, fatigue, night sweats	Very common; raises suspicion of underlying infection
Mucocutaneous (80–90%) (**116–119**)	Oral ulcers	Buccal mucosa, soft palate (may be painless)
	Malar rash	Spares nasolabial fold
	Acute lupus rash	Extensor surfaces, hands, (between joints typical)
	Photosensitivity	Rash, often accompanied by systemic symptoms
	Discoid lupus	Occurs often without systemic disease; predilection for head, neck, and torso; scarring leading to alopecia; pigment changes
	Subacute cutaneous lupus	Erythematous, raised, circumferential; nonscarring; anti-SSA/SSB positive
	Alopecia	Patchy distribution; may be due to discoid lesions/scarring
	Other	Bullous lesions, panniculitis, purpura, secondary Raynaud's, livedo reticularis (aPL antibody)
Musculoskeletal (70–80%) (**120**)	Arthralgias	Nonspecific
	Arthritis	Small joint, symmetric, nonerosive, reversible deformity (Jaccoud's)
	Myalgias	Nonspecific
	Myositis	Uncommon; polymyositis overlap; myopathy can be drug-related (steroids)
Renal (**121**)	Glomerulonephritis (hypertension, hematuria, azotemia)	WHO classification (*Table 41*); often asymptomatic; low C3/C4, anti-dsDNA present
Neurological (**122**)		
• CNS – diffuse	Headache, seizure, aseptic meningitis, psychiatric disease, cognitive dysfunction	Essential to rule out non-SLE etiologies; assessment for aPL antibody syndrome; subtle cognitive dysfunction requiring formal neuropsychiatric testing
• CNS – focal	Stroke, movement disorder, transverse myelitis	
• Peripheral	Mononeuritis, demyelinating syndromes	
Cardiac (**123, 124**)	Pericarditis	Tamponade/constrictive physiology rare; often asymptomatic
	Valvular disease	Libman-Sacks; (aPL antibody)
	Ischemic heart disease	'Precocious'-onset coronary artery disease

(Images overleaf)

(continued)

Table 39 Clinical signs and symptoms in systemic lupus erythematosus (continued)

System	Signs/symptoms	Comments
Pulmonary	Pleurisy/pleuritis	Often small, asymptomatic; exudative
	Pneumonitis	Cause of diffuse alveolar hemorrhage; high mortality
	Thromboembolic disease	aPL antibody
	Pulmonary hypertension	Need to rule out secondary cause (thromboembolic disease)
Hematological	Anemia	Hemolysis (positive Coomb's) *vs.* anemia of chronic disease
	Thrombocytopenia	Similar to idiopathic thrombocytopenic purpura
	Leukopenia	Increased infection risk; lymphopenia characteristic

aPL: antiphospholipid (antibody); CNS: central nervous system; dsDNA: double stranded deoxyribonucleic acid; SLE: systemic lupus erythematosus; WHO: World Health Organization.

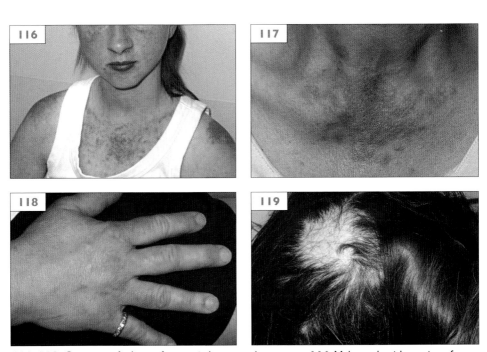

116–119 Cutaneous findings of systemic lupus erythematosus. **116**: Malar rash with sparing of nasolabial folds; **117**: discoid rash; **118**: acute rash on hands, most prominent between joints; **119**: patchy alopecia. (Courtesy of Dr GF Moore.)

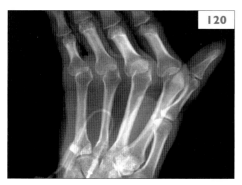

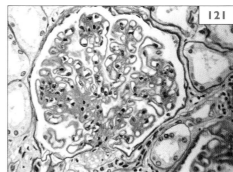

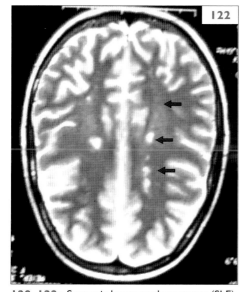

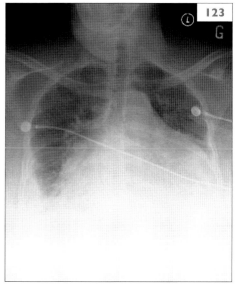

120–122: Systemic lupus erythematosus (SLE). **120:** Hand radiograph in patient with SLE arthropathy; marked deformities that mimic those of rheumatoid arthritis (RA) including ulnar drift of the metacarpophalangeal joints; in contrast to RA, these deformities are reducible in SLE (Jaccoud's arthropathy); note the absence of periarticular erosions. (Courtesy of Dr GF Moore.); **121:** renal histology showing changes of diffuse membranous glomerulonephropathy (WHO Class V). (American College of Rheumatology, with permission.); **122:** brain MRI showing diffuse white matter changes in a patient with systemic lupus erythematosus presenting with acute mental status changes. (Courtesy of Dr GF Moore.)

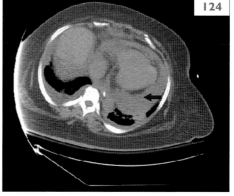

123, 124: Chest radiograph (**123**) and chest CT (**124**) showing large pericardial effusions (arrow) in different patients with systemic lupus erythematosus. (Courtesy of Dr GF Moore.)

further complicated by the fact that 20–30% of patients with SLE are RF-positive. Likewise, CNS lupus may closely mimic multiple sclerosis.

The diagnosis of SLE is based on clinical grounds as there is no single diagnostic test; diagnosis may be guided by disease classification criteria (*Table 38*).

INVESTIGATIONS

- ANA is nonspecific but highly sensitive (>95% with indirect immunofluorescence); newer technologies may lack sensitivity.
- Other autoantibodies (*Table 40*); antibody to extractable nuclear antigens (ENA) is used to evaluate ANA specificity.
- CBC is essential in ruling out hematological involvement, cytopenias; lymphopenia is characteristic of SLE; thrombocytopenia is usually asymptomatic; anemia of chronic disease is common (80%).
- Creatinine and urinalysis to evaluate for renal involvement.
- Complement proteins (C3 and C4 components) are often low with lupus nephritis but may normalize with disease control.
- Kidney biopsy often guides treatment of nephritis; high levels of chronicity suggest poorly responsive disease.
- Other tests (imaging, lumbar puncture, microbiology, other tissue biopsies) are guided by the clinical presentation and evidence of end-organ disease.

HISTOLOGY

Involved tissues, such as the pleura or synovium, may display nonspecific changes of chronic inflammation. Kidney specimens are perhaps the most commonly obtained and show the best characterized findings of SLE, and are used in the World Health Organization (WHO) classification for lupus nephritis (*Table 41*).

PROGNOSIS

There is a bimodal mortality pattern in SLE showing that early mortality is associated with disease activity and infection and late mortality associated with atherosclerotic complications.

Factors associated with higher mortality include lower socioeconomic status, age older than 50 years at the time of diagnosis, male sex, and low complements at the time of diagnosis. Morbidity from treatment or disease is not easy to discern. Infections, coronary artery disease, and osteonecrosis are common sources of morbidity.

MANAGEMENT

The successful management of SLE requires a comprehensive and multidisciplinary approach. Integral to management is patient education, photoprotection, appropriate immunizations, and the identification and treatment of cardiovascular risk factors.

The management of 'mild' or nonmajor organ involvement includes NSAIDs, antimalarials, and glucocorticoids (GCs) (often in low-dose) most commonly.

- NSAIDs are effective for musculoskeletal complaints; caution must be used with renal involvement.
- GCs (prednisone or medrol) are common 'bridge' therapy; lower doses are often adequate for musculoskeletal complaints, higher doses (1.0–1.5 mg/kg/day of prednisone equivalent) are reserved for organ- or life-threatening SLE; adverse effects are common and are dose-related.
- Antimalarials (HCQ) are widely used for the musculoskeletal, cutaneous, and constitutional symptoms; they may reduce flare frequency and improve overall survival but have slow onset of action. Retinal toxicity is rare (routine ophthalmologic evaluation is required). Immunomodulating, immunosuppressive, or cytotoxic drugs are often needed for moderate to severe lupus with major organ involvement:
- Azathioprine (AZA) is a purine analog, and inhibits nucleic acid synthesis; it is an oral therapy, at a dose of 1–2 mg/kg per day; severe drug–drug interaction with allopurinol occurs; side-effects include GI- and myelosuppression (CBC monitoring is essential).

Table 40 Autoantibodies in systemic lupus erythematosus (SLE), clinical associations, and disease specificity

Autoantibody	Clinical association	SLE specificity
Anti-dsDNA	Lupus nephritis	✓
Anti-Sm	None	✓
Anti-RNP	Raynaud's, ILD, PHTN	
Antiphospholipid	Clotting disorders	
Antiribosomal P	Diffuse central nervous system disease and psychiatric disease	✓
Anti-SSA/Ro	Dry eyes and mouth, SCLE, neonatal lupus, and photosensitivity	
Anti-SSB/La	Dry eyes and mouth, SCLE, neonatal lupus, and photosensitivity	
Histone	SLE and drug-induced lupus	

dsDNA: double-stranded deoxyribonucleic acid; ILD: interstitial lung disease; PHTN: pulmonary hypertension; RNP: ribonucleoprotein; Sm: Smith; SCLE: subacute cutaneous lupus erythematosus.

Table 41 World Health Organization classification of lupus nephritis

Class	Pattern	Site of immune complexes	Clinical clues
I	Minimal mesangial	Mesangial	Bland sediment, normal complements and negative anti-dsDNA antibody
II	Proliferative mesangial	Mesangial	Bland sediment with normal complements and negative anti-dsDNA antibody
III	Focal	Mesangial, subendothelial, ± subepithelial	Active sediment, proteinuria, with low complements and high anti-dsDNA antibody
IV	Diffuse	Mesangial, subendothelial, ± subepithelial	Active sediment, proteinuria, with low complements and high anti-dsDNA antibody
V	Membranous	Mesangial, subepithelial	Bland sediment with significant proteinuria, normal complements, and variable anti-dsDNA antibody
VI	Advanced sclerosing	None	High serum creatinine with evidence of end-stage renal disease

dsDNA: double stranded deoxyribonucleic acid.

- Cyclophosphamide (CTX) is an alkylating agent given as daily oral or intermittent (monthly) intravenous therapy; it requires close clinical and laboratory surveillance.
- Mycophenolate mofetil (MMF) has an important role in lupus nephritis.
- Other immunomodulating agents that work through B cell depletion (e.g. rituximab) and other agents targeting lymphocyte expression/ function are under active investigation.

Drug-induced lupus

DEFINITION

Drug-induced lupus (DIL) refers to the development of a lupus-like syndrome following the exposure to select drugs, which classically has involved the use of procainamide and hydralazine, but more recently has included the use of biologic therapies and minocycline.

EPIDEMIOLOGY AND ETIOLOGY

There are an estimated 15 000 to 30 000 cases of DIL per year in the US. It is equally common in men and women with the exception of minocycline-induced lupus, which occurs more commonly in young woman. Approximately 10% of SLE cases are estimated to be 'drug-induced'.

A variety of drugs have been identified as being associated with DIL (*Table 42*). Agents associated with the highest risk of DIL include:

- Procainamide (up to 15–20%).
- Hydralazine (up to 7–13%).
- Penicillamine.

DIL risks for other agents are estimated to be two per 1000 for those taking antitumor necrosis factor (anti-TNF)-α drugs and five per 10 000 of those taking minocycline.

Medications can induce different autoantibodies such as ANA and anti-neutrophil cytoplasmic antibody (ANCA), but it is not an indication to stop treatment if clinical features are absent. Almost 90% of patients treated with procainamide develop detectable ANA, but only 20% develop the features of lupus. This is the case for many medications.

PATHOGENESIS

The mechanisms involved in DIL remain uncertain with various theories developed regarding its pathogenesis. Although not necessarily generalizable to other agents associated with DIL, drugs including procainamide, chlorpromazine, and quinidine lead to the formation of ANA antibodies targeting histone complexes.

CLINICAL HISTORY AND PHYSICAL EXAMINATION

DIL typically has its onset months to years after the initiation of the offending agent. SLE flares in a patient with established disease can occur shortly after exposure to some drugs that are also associated with DIL. Signs and symptoms of DIL include skin rash, photosensitivity, arthralgias and arthritis (**125**), pleural and pericardial effusions (**126**), lymphadenopathy, and splenomegaly. Pleuropulmonary disease is prominent, particularly with procainamide. 'End-organ' damage including hematologic abnormalities, kidney disease, and CNS involvement are uncommon and their presence should underscore the possibility of SLE.

DIL can also present as predominant cutaneous forms including subacute cutaneous lupus erythematosus (SCLE) and chronic cutaneous lupus erythematosus (CCLE).

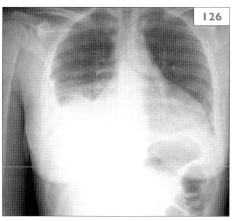

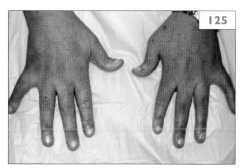

125 Joint involvement with arthralgias and arthritis affecting primarily small joints of the hands can be presenting features of drug-induced lupus. (Courtesy of Dr GF Moore.)

126 Chest radiograph showing large pleural and pericardial effusions in a patient with drug-induced lupus. (Courtesy of Dr GF Moore.)

Table 42 Drugs classes and agents associated with drug-induced lupus

Anticonvulsants	Antihypertensives	Other
Carbamazepine, hydantoins, ethosuximide, primidone, trimethadione	Hydralazine, methyldopa, captopril, hydrochlorothiazide	Penicillamine, chlorpromazine, phenylbutazone, thiazides, oral contraceptive pills, levodopa, lithium carbonate, HMG-CoA reductase agents, TNF-α inhibitors, interferon-α, glyburide, terbinafine, ticlopidine, docetaxel, statins (lovastatin, simvastatin, atorvastatin), gemfibrosil, griseofulvin
Antiarrhythmics	Beta-adrenergic blockers	**Biologic agents**
Procainamide, quinidine, amiodarone	Labetalol, acebutol, pindolol	TNF-α inhibitors, interferon-α, interleukins
Antibiotics	**Antithyroidals**	
Minocycline, isoniazide, sulfasalzine, penicillin, streptomycin, sulfonamides, griseofulvin, nitrofurantoin	Propiothiouracil, methylthiouracil	

TNF: tumor necrosis factor.

Antihypertensives and antifungal drugs are the most common drugs implicated in SCLE (associated with anti-Ro/La antibody).

DIFFERENTIAL DIAGNOSIS
The differential diagnosis is often determined by the primary presenting signs and symptoms, and may include other entities causing rash and/or inflammatory arthritis. Other forms of 'idiopathic' lupus (SLE, discoid lupus, SCLE, and neonatal lupus) must be excluded.

There are no definitive diagnostic criteria, but the presence of DIL should be suspected in a patient presenting with characteristic clinical features who has been taking an associated agent (*Table 42*) for at least 1 month. Additional findings of ANA positivity (antihistone antibody) in the absence of other autoantibodies is suggestive.

INVESTIGATIONS
The laboratory profile of a patient with DIL may help distinguish the syndrome from spontaneous SLE. While ANA are typically present, serum complements are usually normal and antibodies to double stranded deoxyribonucleic acid (ds-DNA) are usually absent (although may be observed in some forms of DIL including that associated with anti-TNF, interferon [IFN], and minocycline).

Infrequent in SLE, some forms of DIL (e.g. minocycline) are associated with concomitant hepatitis resulting in elevated liver transaminases. Antihistone antibodies are present in more than 95% of cases, recognizing that these are positive in many patients with SLE. Anti-ds-DNA antibodies are often present in disease associated with use of anti-TNF agents and interferon-α and typically absent with drug-induced disease with other agents. Other ANA-related autoantibody (anti-RNP, anti-Smith) are typically absent in DIL.

Other laboratory tests may be necessary to evaluate for the possibility of evidence of 'end-organ disease' more typical of SLE:
• CBC with differential to detect cytopenias.
• Urinalysis to examine for proteinuria and active urinary sediment.
• Serum creatinine to evaluate for azotemia.
Chest radiograph and/or echocardiography may be needed to evaluate for evidence of pleuropericardial involvement.

HISTOLOGY
Although biopsy is only rarely indicated in DIL, involved tissues typically show changes consistent with lupus (see p. 126).

PROGNOSIS
Outcomes related to DIL are usually excellent following withdrawal of the offending agent. Long-term morbidity and mortality related to DIL are rare.

MANAGEMENT
Discontinuation of the offending medication typically leads to resolution of symptoms within weeks to months; DIL-related autoantibody may persist even after clinical resolution. Symptomatic management, including NSAIDs and low-dose GCs may be needed for debilitating symptoms in some cases.

Antiphospholipid antibody syndrome

DEFINITION
Antiphospholipid antibody syndrome (APS) is an autoimmune disease that is characterized clinically by vascular thrombosis and pregnancy loss, and serologically by the presence of circulating antiphospholipid antibodies (aPL).

EPIDEMIOLOGY AND ETIOLOGY
Low-titer, transient aPL occur in up to 10% of the normal population, but moderate to high titer aPL occur in less than 1%. The prevalence of aPL increases with age. These antibodies are also seen concomitantly with other rheumatic diseases: 10–40% of SLE patients and 20% of RA patients have positive aPL. Asymptomatic aPL-positive patients have a 0–4% annual risk of thrombosis. Importantly, 10% of first-stroke victims have aPL, and this increases to 29% in young patients. Up to 20% of women with three or more fetal losses have positive aPL, and 14% of patients with recurrent deep vein thrombosis (DVT) have aPL.

Pathologic autoimmune aPL most likely results from cross-reactivity with a common infection in a genetically susceptible person. A variety of bacterial, viral, and parasitic infections have been associated with aPL. In addition, drugs (chlorpromazine, procainamide, quinidine, and phenytoin) and malignancies (lymphoproliferative disorders) can also induce aPL.

PATHOGENESIS
The aPLs are a family of autoantibodies directed against plasma proteins that are bound to negatively charged phospholipids. *In vitro*, aPL primarily target the phospholipid-binding plasma protein β2-glycoprotein-I. The most commonly detected subgroups of aPL are lupus anticoagulant (LAC) antibodies, anticardiolipin (aCL) antibodies, and anti-β2 glycoprotein I (β2-GP-I) antibodies.

Many theories have been offered to explain how aPL triggers thrombosis. The leading theory proposes that aPL induces tissue factor in endothelial cells leading to monocyte and complement activation, platelet aggregation, and the expression of endothelial cell adhesion receptor. Animal models further support the central importance of complement activation in APS pathology.

CLINICAL HISTORY AND PHYSICAL EXAMINATION
Clinical manifestations in APS range from asymptomatic aPL positivity to catastrophic thromboses.
- Venous thrombosis: DVT and pulmonary embolus are most common; can occur in unusual anatomic locations (renal vein, Budd–Chiari syndrome, portal, mesenteric and adrenal veins).
- Arterial occlusion: Stroke and transient ischemic attack are the most common types; peripheral/ophthalmic arteries may be affected.
- Recurrent fetal loss/other obstetric manifestations (pre-eclampsia/eclampsia, hemolysis, elevated liver enzymes, and low platelet count [HELLP] syndrome).

Many patients may have miscellaneous manifestations although not specific for APS. These include:
- Hematologic: Thrombocytopenia, Coombs-positive hemolytic anemia.
- Cutaneous: Livedo reticularis (**127**).

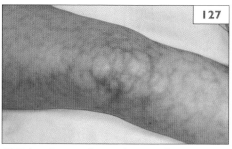

127 Livedo reticularis is the most frequent dermatological manifestation observed in a patient with antiphospholipid antibody syndrome. (Courtesy of Dr GF Moore.)

- Other neurological manifestations: Cognitive impairment, headache.
- Renal: Renal insufficiency, proteinuria, hypertension.
- Cardiac: Valvular lesions (aseptic vegetations, thickening, dysfunction – mitral and/or aortic insufficiency), myocardial microthrombosis, intracardiac thrombi, ventricular dysfunction.
- Musculoskeletal: Avascular necrosis.
  Catastrophic APS (CAPS) is a rare, abrupt, life-threatening complication. CAPS is characterized by rapidly progressive multiorgan failure due to predominantly small vessel thrombi in patients with aPLs. Definite CAPS is defined as evidence of involvement of three or more organs in <1 week with confirmatory pathology and laboratory confirmation of the presence of aPLs.

DIFFERENTIAL DIAGNOSIS
- Presence of aPL: aPLs occur transiently sometimes following infection (immunoglobulin [Ig]M >>> IgG); transient low-titer aPL is considered inconclusive for diagnosis; infection-induced aPL is usually not pathogenic (hepatitis C virus [HCV], and human immunodeficiency virus [HIV] infections are possible exceptions).
- Recurrent pregnancy loss: 5–21% of women with recurrent pregnancy losses and 0.5–2% of normal pregnant women have aPL; fetal loss is more commonly due to APS after 10 weeks' gestation.
- Arterial and venous thrombosis: Broad differential including alternative causes of thromboembolic disease (other hypercoagulable states; i.e. protein C/S deficiency, Factor V Leiden, and so on).
  The diagnosis of APS is made using a positive serologic test in the appropriate clinical context. Classification criteria have been developed for research purposes, but can be useful as a clinical guide (*Table 43*).

Table 43 Revised Sapporo Classification Criteria for antiphospholipid antibody syndrome

Clinical criteria

Vascular thrombosis including one or more clinical episodes of arterial, venous, or small-vessel thrombosis in any tissue or organ

Pregnancy morbidity: (a) one or more unexplained deaths of a morphologically normal fetus during or after 10th week of gestation; (b) one or more premature births of a morphologically normal neonate before the 34th week of gestation because of eclampsia or severe pre-eclampsia or severe placental insufficiency; or (c) three or more unexplained consecutive spontaneous abortions before the 10th week of gestation, with anatomic, hormonal, and chromosomal abnormalities excluded

Laboratory criteria

Lupus anticoagulant present in plasma on two or more occasions at least 12 weeks apart

Anticardiolipin antibody of IgG or IgM in serum or plasma, in medium or high titer (>40 GPL or MPL, or >99th percentile) on two or more occasions at least 12 weeks apart by ELISA

Anti–ß2-glycoprotein I antibody of IgG or IgM isotype in serum or plasma (in titer >99th percentile) present on two or more occasions at least 12 weeks apart, measured by ELISA

APS is present if at least one of the clinical criteria and one of the laboratory criteria are met. ELISA: enzyme-linked immunosorbent assay; GPL: IgG anticardiolipin antibody unit*; Ig: immunoglobulin; MPL: IgM anticardiolipin antibody unit*.

*correlated from an original index sample.

INVESTIGATIONS

- LAC
  Step 1: Prolonged coagulation time (activated partial thromboplastin time [aPTT], dilute Russell viper venom time [dRVTT]).
  Step 2: Confirmation by failure to correct prolonged coagulation time by mixing the patient plasma with normal plasma (1:1); note that coagulation time corrects if originally prolonged due to factor deficiency.
  Step 3: Further confirmation of LAC via shortening or correction of the prolonged coagulation time after addition of excess phospholipids or platelets that have been frozen and thawed.
  Step 4: Ruling out other coagulopathies with the use of specific factor assays if the confirmatory test is negative or if a specific factor inhibitor is suspected.
- aCL antibody IgG, IgM by enzyme-linked immunosorbent assay (ELISA); diagnosis requires moderate to high-titer; highly sensitive but not specific; repeated in 12 weeks; consider testing IgA aCL if other tests are negative with high clinical suspicion.
- Anti-β2-GP-I antibody IgG, IgM by ELISA; more specific than aCL.
- Other tests: Other tests may be helpful in evaluating for overlapping rheumatic condition (ANA, RF) and evidence of end-organ involvement (creatinine, urinalysis); CBC is essential in evaluating for cytopenias; lower extremity Doppler, computed tomography (CT) angiogram, and alternative imaging techniques may be needed to rule out thromboembolic disease (**128**).

HISTOLOGY

Histological examination of the vessels, skin, kidney, or other involved tissues may demonstrate thrombus formation without surrounding inflammation, acute and chronic endothelial injury and its sequelae, with recanalization in late lesions.

PROGNOSIS

During long-term follow-up in APS, serious morbidity and disability can occur, although in an unpredictable fashion. Patients with APS and a history of pregnancy-related morbidity are at higher risk for future vascular thrombosis. CAPS recurrence is unusual and patients who survive often experience a stable clinical course with continued anticoagulation. Serious perioperative complications may occur despite prophylaxis, and patients with APS are at additional risk for thrombosis when they undergo surgery.

MANAGEMENT

- Asymptomatic aPL: Current evidence does not support the effectiveness of aspirin or other treatment modalities in primary prevention.
- aPL in pregnancy:
  - Low aCL, no previous loss – no treatment.
  - + aPL and single pregnancy loss at <10 week – no treatment or low-dose aspirin.
  - + aPL and >2 early or >1 late loss, no thrombosis – low-dose aspirin and prophylactic low-molecular weight heparin (LMWH) throughout the pregnancy; discontinued 6–12 weeks postpartum.
  - Thrombosis regardless of pregnancy history – therapeutic heparin and low-dose aspirin throughout pregnancy; warfarin given postpartum.

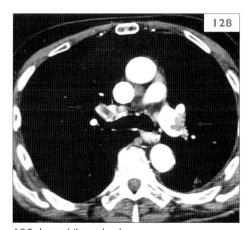

128 Large bilateral pulmonary thromboembolism demonstrated on CT angiogram (arrows); pulmonary embolism can be the initial clinical manifestation of antiphospholipid antibody syndrome (Courtesy of Dr GF Moore.)

- Venous thrombosis: Anticoagulation (heparin overlapped with warfarin); moderate-intensity warfarin (international normalized ratio [INR] 2–3) for secondary prophylaxis; duration of therapy is uncertain but patients are often treated indefinitely due to a high risk for recurrent thrombosis.
- Arterial thrombosis: Warfarin (INR 2–3) indefinitely; there is ongoing debate on the intensity of anticoagulation (moderate *vs.* high-intensity).
- Recurrent thrombosis: INR must be at therapeutic levels; factor II should be checked at the time of the event with INR (therapeutic INR may not be *effective* INR in all patients with LAC); other treatment modalities including higher-dose warfarin, unfractionated or LMWH, adding low-dose aspirin, adding other therapies (HCQ, statin) should be considered.
- CAPS: Precipitating factors should be treated; supportive care and anticoagulation given; pulse high-dose GCs, intravenous immunoglobulin (IVIG), plasma exchange with fresh frozen plasma (FFP) and, in select situations, other modalities such as CTX or rituximab should all be considered.

Polymyositis and dermatomyositis

DEFINITION
Polymyositis (PM) is a chronic idiopathic form of inflammatory myopathy, leading to progressive muscle weakness. Dermatomyositis (DM) is a closely related disorder characterized by inflammatory changes in both the muscle and skin.

EPIDEMIOLOGY AND ETIOLOGY
PM and DM are relatively uncommon CTDs, with an incidence of approximately 0.5–1.0 cases per 100 000 patient-years of follow-up. PM/DM affects all age groups, including children (with a disease incidence approximately half of that seen in adults). In adults, disease incidence increases with age with a slight female to male predominance (~2:1). PM/DM has been reported to be more common in African-Americans than Caucasians, but studies examining racial/ethnic differences in disease risk are limited. Both PM and DM have been reported to co-occur with malignancy, most commonly adenocarcinomas or other solid tumors. This risk appears to be more pronounced with DM compared with PM.

The etiology of PM/DM is not well understood. In contrast with other CTDs, PM/DM does not display significant familial clustering, suggesting that environmental factors may play an important (yet ill-defined) role in triggering the disease. Environmental factors speculated to play a role in PM/DM include select infections (toxoplasmosis, Epstein–Barr virus, coxsackie virus, and mycoplasma) in addition to exposure to other exogenous toxins/chemicals. As with other CTDs, there is speculation that exposure to an environmental trigger leads to 'neoantigen' presentation and secondary inflammation (characterized by lymphocytic infiltration of involved muscles), possibly through 'molecular mimicry'.

PATHOGENESIS
Although incompletely understood, it has been hypothesized that an initial muscle injury leads to the presentation of an 'autoantigen'. This antigen is thought to be processed and presented to T cells in the context of MHC class I. Once activated, T cells in PM/DM synthesize interferon-γ, which in turn leads to increased expression of proinflammatory cytokines including IL-1 and TNF.

CLINICAL HISTORY AND PHYSICAL EXAMINATION

PM/DM generally result in insidious and progressive muscle weakness, often in the absence of significant pain. Muscle weakness is typically most prominent in proximal muscle groups, leading to problems with activities such as climbing/descending stairs or rising from a seated position. Although distal muscle weakness can occur with disease progression, a suggestive history (e.g. weakness in grip, dropping things) should prompt an assessment of alternative etiologies (see below). Skin involvement or rash in DM can occur at any time point relative to the onset of muscle weakness. Generalized symptoms may include progressive fatigue, fevers, RP, and weight loss. In rare circumstances, typical DM skin involvement can occur in the absence of apparent myopathy (so-called 'DM sine myositis'). Other clinical history should be sought that could be indicative of co-occurring malignancy or extraskeletal muscle or other end-organ involvement: arthralgias related to an inflammatory arthritis; dysphagia due to esophageal involvement; dyspnea and/or dry cough related to either pulmonary (e.g. interstitial lung disease [ILD]) or cardiac involvement (pericarditis or myocarditis).

A thorough and systematic examination may reveal:
- Symmetric weakness most prominent in proximal muscle groups.
- Skin involvement suggestive of DM:
  - Gottron's papules (pathognomonic of DM); palpable erythematous lesions over the extensor surfaces of the hands (over metacarpal–phalangeal [MCP] and proximal interphalangeal [PIP] joints) (**129**), elbows, or knees.
  - Gottron's sign: nonpalpable rash, similar distribution to Gottron's papules.
  - Heliotrope rash (**130**); occurs around the eyes, variable in appearance.
  - Erythroderma.
  - V-sign (**131**), shawl sign, and 'mechanics hands' (**132**).
  - Calcinosis (more common in juvenile DM).
- Extramuscular or end-organ involvement: arrhythmia or gallop suggestive of cardiac involvement; lung crackles suggestive of pulmonary disease.

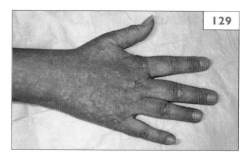

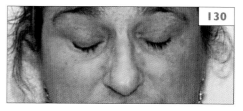

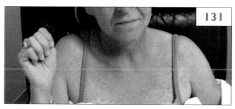

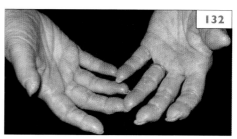

129–132 Skin findings characteristic of dermatomyositis. **129**: Gottron's papules, consisting of palpable erythematous plaques over the extensor surfaces of the hands; **130**: heliotrope rash; **131**: the V-sign; **132**: mechanic's hands. (Courtesy of Dr GF Moore.)

DIFFERENTIAL DIAGNOSIS

The differential diagnosis for inflammatory myopathy and proximal muscle weakness is quite extensive (*Table 44*). Inclusion body myositis (IBM) is a rare form of inflammatory myopathy that shares many clinical similarities with PM (progressive weakness, increased incidence with age). In contrast to PM/DM, IBM typically results in 'lower grade' elevations in muscle enzymes, can be less symmetric, and involves distal muscle groups. Its onset may also be more insidious (years *vs.* months) and it is far more refractory to treatment (with a resulting poor prognosis) compared with PM/DM. Muscle biopsy (see below) is critical in distinguishing IBM from PM/DM. Criteria for the diagnosis of an inflammatory myopathy are:

1 Symmetric weakness, usually progressive, involving the proximal muscles.
2 Muscle biopsy indicative of inflammatory myopathy (see below).
3 Elevation of muscle enzymes on laboratory examination (see below).
4 EMG findings suggestive of inflammatory myopathy (see below).
5 Characteristic skin findings of DM (e.g. heliotrope rash, Gottron's papules, or Gottron's sign).

Table 44 Differential diagnosis for inflammatory myopathy/progressive proximal muscle weakness

Connective tissue diseases	Inheritable disorders
Overlap syndromes (systemic lupus erythematosus, scleroderma)	Mitochondrial myopathies (e.g. McCardle's)
Sarcoidosis	Muscular dystrophies
Inclusion body myositis	
Infections	**Neuropathy/neuromuscular disease**
Viral (hepatitis, influenza, coxsackie)	Guillain–Barré
Bacterial	Autoimmune polyneuropathy
Fungal/protozoal	Amyotrophic lateral sclerosis
	Myasthenia gravis
	Eaton–Lambert
Toxins/medications	**Endocrine**
Lipid-lowering agents (e.g. statins)	Hypo- or hyperthyroidism
Ethanol	Diabetes
Colchicine	Acromegaly
Hydroxychloroquine	Cushing's or Addison's syndrome
Antipsychotics (malignant hyperthermia)	Hypokalemia
Cocaine/amphetamines	Hypophosphotemia
L-tryptophan (eosinophilia myalgia syndrome)	Hyocalcemia
Trauma/overuse syndromes	Hypomagnesemia

These criteria are based on the assumption that alternative causes of myopathy have been ruled out (*Table 44*). Patients are said to have 'definite' inflammatory myopathy if criteria 1–4 are present (1–5 for DM); 'probable' if three of the first four criteria are met (plus No. 5 for DM); or 'possible' if two of the first four criteria are met (plus No. 5 for DM).

INVESTIGATIONS
Laboratory
- Muscle enzymes: Although not disease specific, serum muscle enzymes elevated in the context of PM/DM include:
  - Creatine kinase: often >2-times upper normal.
  - Lactate dehydrogenase.
  - Aldolase.
  - Aspartate aminotransferase.

Muscle enzymes are helpful in following treatment effectiveness and elevations may actually precede clinical symptoms. In very rare cases, patients with active PM/DM may have normal muscle enzyme levels. Marked muscle breakdown due to inflammation may result in increased myoglobin in serum and urine (the latter resulting in heme-positive urine dipstick without demonstrable red blood cells).
- Acute phase reactants: ESR and C-reactive protein (CRP) are often normal; marked elevations should raise suspicion for other causes of inflammation (infection).
- Autoantibodies:
  - ANAs: suggestive but not diagnostic of an underlying CTD (i.e. PM/DM); positive in 60–90%
  - Anti-tRNA synthetases: seen in a subset of patients (~25% of DM); disproportionate occurrence of ILD, mechanic's hands, and RP (anti-Jo-1 antibody is the most commonly measured antisynthetase antibody).
  - Anti-RNP: seen in context of MCTD.
  - Antisignal recognition protein antibody: characterized by necrotizing acute-onset polymyositis, cardiac involvement, and poor treatment response.
  - Anti-Mi-2: classic DM; excellent treatment response.
- EMG and magnetic resonance imaging (MRI): The characteristic 'triad' of EMG findings in PM/DM include the presence of 1) short, small, low-amplitude polyphasic motor units; 2) fibrillation potentials; and 3) atypical high-frequency repetitive discharges.

EMG is typically done unilaterally in upper and lower extremities as needle artifact can interfere with biopsy and histological interpretation. Tests of nerve conduction velocity (NCVs) performed in conjunction with EMG are helpful in ruling out a neuropathic etiology.

MRI short T1 inversion recovery (STIR) may be an alternative means for detecting inflammatory muscle changes. MRI STIR reveals marked enhancement in involved muscles (**133**). As with muscle enzyme tests, neither EMG nor MRI STIR are by themselves diagnostic, but are most helpful in identifying optimal sites for biopsy.
- Muscle biopsy: Most often done in the quadriceps or deltoid muscles. Biopsy is critical in excluding alternative diagnoses such as IBM or sarcoidosis (see 'Histology' below). EMG/MRI are helpful in optimizing biopsy yield.
- Skin biopsy: Skin biopsy may be useful with atypical presentations (e.g. DM sine myositis) and may be particularly helpful in ruling out alternative causes of rash (See Histology below).
- Other: Other laboratory or imaging tests may be needed to rule out alternative diagnoses (*Table 44*), the co-occurrence of malignancy, or if the history and/or physical examination suggest other organ system involvement. Given associations of PM/DM with malignancy, age-appropriate cancer screening should be performed. Increasingly, standard-of-care includes imaging of the chest, abdomen, and pelvis in evaluating for occult malignancy. Patients presenting with dyspnea or chronic cough may need pulmonary and/or cardiac evaluations (chest radiograph, pulmonary function tests, electrocardiogram [ECG], echocardiogram). Patients with marked dysphagia may require further endoscopic examination.

HISTOLOGY
There are subtle differences in histopathologic findings in PM *vs.* DM. Involved muscle in PM typically shows focal endomysial mononuclear cell infiltration while muscle tissue in DM displays

perivascular and interstitial inflammation. As detailed above, histopathology is essential in ruling out alternative etiologies. IBM is characterized by the presence of 'rimmed vacuoles' (seen best with electron microscopy) or typical nuclear or cytoplasmic microtubular filaments that can be seen using light microscopy.

PROGNOSIS

Overall survival in PM/DM has improved, now exceeding 80–90%. Poor prognostic factors include: co-occurrence of malignancy, older age at onset, female gender, severe end-organ involvement (dysphagia, ILD, cardiomyopathy), and the presence of antisynthetase or antisignal recognition particle (anti-SRP) antibody. Given its poor response to therapy, IBM has a particularly poor prognosis.

MANAGEMENT
Primary therapy includes

- Systemic GCs (e.g. prednisone, 1–2 mg/kg/day); typically maintained, if possible, until normalization of muscle enzyme concentrations; gradually tapered over the course of several months to years.
- Methotrexate (MTX) or AZA; used concomitantly with GCs; may allow for more rapid GC tapering.
- Physical therapy and sun avoidance for those with photosensitivity.
  Secondary therapy involves:
- HCQ: possible utility in skin disease although rarely patients may experience an exacerbation with its use.
- CTX: indications include ILD or overlapping vasculitis.
- IVIG (0.5–1.0 g/kg/day): sometimes used as induction therapy in severe or refractory disease; possible role in IBM.
- Second-line treatments used with limited data include cyclosporine, tacrolimus, MMF, anti-TNF agents, and B cell depletion (rituximab).

Disease flares or recurrence can occur during GC tapering and/or withdrawal. Disease flare can be confused with steroid-induced myopathy, distinguished from active inflammatory myopathy by the lack of muscle enzyme elevation and normal MRI STIR. Weakness in the context of PM/DM treatment due to flare must also be distinguished from weakness caused from chronic damage or scarring. With chronic damage or scarring, muscle enzymes are typically normal (or even reduced), while EMG and MRI fail to show evidence of active myopathy.

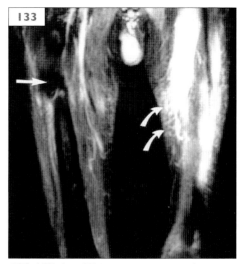

133 MRI short T1 inversion recovery showing areas of enhancement consistent with active myositis. (Courtesy of Dr GF Moore.)

Systemic sclerosis (scleroderma)

DEFINITION

Systemic sclerosis (scleroderma) (SSc) is a multisystem CTD resulting in diffuse fibrosis of the skin, internal organs, and connective tissues. The course is chronic and there is no cure.

There are several scleroderma spectrum disorders, outlined in *Table 45*. These disorders range from a small area of skin involvement to diffuse skin and multiorgan disease. This chapter focuses primarily on diffuse SSc.

EPIDEMIOLOGY AND ETIOLOGY

Scleroderma has a worldwide distribution. In the US, the estimated incidence is 9–19 cases/million/year and the estimated prevalence is 28–253 cases per million. SSc affects women three to seven times more commonly than men, and the age of onset is classically between 45 and 65 years old. SSc affects all races, but in African-Americans the disease usually occurs earlier and has a worse prognosis.

Table 45 Scleroderma spectrum of diseases

Limited cutaneous SSc	Skin thickening limited distally to elbows and knees, and may involve the neck and face. PHTN may occur
Diffuse cutaneous SSc	Diffuse skin thickening, including the trunk, extremities and face. Internal organ involvement is common
CREST syndrome	A limited form of SSc with prominent calcinosis, RP, esophageal dysmotility, sclerodactyly and telangectasia. PHTN can occur
Overlap SSc	SSc disease manifestations in coexisting with other rheumatic disease: SLE, myositis, or RA
SSc sine scleroderma	RP and other clinical and serological manifestations of SSc, but lacking the skin changes
Morphea	Localized area of skin involvement, but can become generalized
Linear scleroderma	Linear, band-like, sclerotic lesions which often follow a dermatome. Problematic when occurring over a joint line
Coup de sabre	Linear SSc occurring on the face or scalp. Underlying bone and brain tissue may be involved (**134, 135**)

CREST: calcinosis, Raynaud's phenomenon, esophageal dysmotility, sclerodactyly, telangectasia; PHTN: pulmonary arterial hypertension; RA: rheumatoid arthritis; RP: Raynaud's phenomenon; SSc: scleroderma; SLE: systemic lupus erythematosus.

(Images overleaf)

The etiology of SSc remains elusive. There are genetic factors involved, but the method of inheritance is still under investigation and likely to be highly complex. There have also been suggested links between viral infections, environmental exposures, drugs, and radiation with the development of SSc. To date, no clear explanation for the development of SSc exists.

PATHOGENESIS

There are three aberrant pathways involved in the development of SSc: vasculopathy, inflammation, and fibrosis. Early in the development of SSc, inflammation is present in many organs. The vascular derangements in SSc occur early and may be the initiating event. The trigger for endothelial cell damage is unknown, but once initiated, ensues in a wide-spread fashion. Early vascular changes include a bland intimal proliferation, impaired fibrinolysis and platelet aggregation. This continues with eventual fibrin deposition, resulting in luminal occlusion and tissue hypoxia.

The inflammatory component of SSc involves both the cellular and humoral arms of the immune system. Macrophages, lymphocytes, eosinophils, mast cells, and natural killer (NK) cells are all found in the perivascular areas of involved tissue before there is evidence of fibrosis. Macrophages produce transforming growth factor (TGF)-β, among other proinflammatory cytokines, which is a potent inducer of fibroblast activation and collagen synthesis. B cells are involved and produce several disease specific auto-antibodies (*Table 46, overleaf*).

SSc is typified by aberrant and dysregulated tissue fibrosis. TGF-β and other cytokines, chemokines and growth factors that promote fibrosis are elevated in SSc. Ultimately, the SSc fibroblast becomes phenotypically altered so that it remains active, despite the presence of inhibitory signals. The end result is widespread, progressive fibrosis of multiple organs and connective tissues.

CLINICAL HISTORY

The earliest features of SSc to manifest are usually in the skin. RP, a well-demarcated, triphasic color (white, then blue, then red) change in the hands and feet provoked by cold or emotional stress, is almost universally present (**136**). Frequently, the hands, wrists, and lower extremities will have edema which then evolves to include inflammatory changes and pruritis. Eventually, involved skin becomes fibrotic and hide bound, but may soften as time goes on. Pigmentary changes (hypo- and hyperpigmentation) may occur. Chronic digital ischemia results in distal ulcerations and tissue resorption. Telangectasia is also a common finding on the skin and mucous membranes (**137**).

Vascular changes also include nailfold capillary changes and vascular ectasia of the stomach (**138**). Pulmonary hypertension (PHTN) can also be present, but is more common in the limited forms of SSc. In addition to vascular changes in the GI tract, dysmotility can affect the entire tract. This results in gastroesophageal reflux, with esophageal strictures and Barrett's esophagus. Postprandial bloating and nausea are a result of delayed gastric emptying. Small intestinal dysmotility results in bacterial overgrowth, which can lead to malabsorption, weight loss, and diarrhea. Intestinal ileus may also be problematic. Large bowel involvement includes constipation, large mouth diverticuli, sigmoid volvulus, and anorectal incontinence. Although the liver and pancreas are usually spared, primary biliary cirrhosis can be seen with SSc, but usually is seen the limited subtypes.

Although arthralgia can be a common complaint, frank arthritis is uncommon. Fibrosis of the connective tissues around joints can lead to contractures and friction rubs. Bony resorption of the distal fingers (acro-osteolysis), ribs, and mandible may occur from hypoxemia from vascular changes.

In addition to the myopathy seen in the GI tract, both skeletal and cardiac muscle involvement is seen in SSc. Skeletal muscle changes can include a fibrotic or an inflammatory myopathy. Cardiac muscle involvement is likely underrecognized and has a major impact on survival. Changes in the cardiac muscle may include ischemia, myocarditis, or fibrosis.

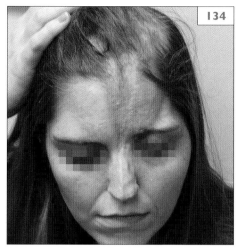

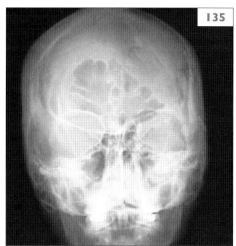

134, 135 A patient with coup de sabre scleroderma; the corresponding radiograph (135) shows involvement of underlying tissues. (Courtesy of Dr GF Moore.)

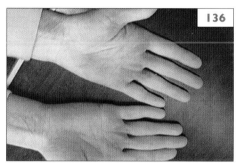

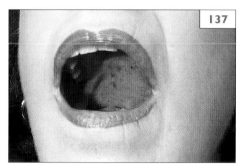

136 An episode of Raynaud's phenomenon manifest by well-demarcated areas of white in multiple fingers, often followed by cyanosis (blue discoloration) followed by hyperemia (red discoloration). (Courtesy of Dr GF Moore.)

137 Telangiectasia of the oral mucosa in a patient with scleroderma. (Courtesy of Dr GF Moore.)

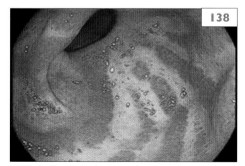

138 Endoscopic findings showing diffuse vascular ectasia of the stomach in a patient with diffuse scleroderma. (Courtesy of American College of Rheumatology.)

The pulmonary parenchyma and vasculature can also be involved. Parenchymal inflammation and interstitial changes can progress to an irreversible pulmonary fibrosis (**139**). PHTN may also result from this fibrotic process, with loss of vascular beds, or may occur more directly from intimal changes in the pulmonary arterial bed. Aspiration pneumonitis, pleural effusions, bronchiectasis, and lung cancer are also reported.

The renal vasculature is also affected and SSc renal crisis is one of the most feared complications of this disease. Usually occurring within the first year of disease, renal crisis presents with accelerated hypertension with microangiopathic hemolysis and a decline in renal function. Without treatment, renal failure can result. Nerve entrapment may occur from perineural tissue fibrosis. Fibrosis also leads to the loss of exocrine functions of the skin and mucus membranes and can result in dryness and sicca symptoms. The course of SSc can be variable in the individual patient, but in general, those with diffuse disease manifest skin and internal organ changes within the first 18 months of disease.

PHYSICAL EXAMINATION

Because of the diffuse nature of SSc, a very thorough physical examination should be performed. Physical examination findings in SSc include:

- Early edematous changes in the skin which progress to a woody indurated skin with pigmentary changes; this may result in the inability to flatten the hands against each other (the so-called 'prayer sign') (**140**).
- Nailfold capillary dilation and 'drop-offs' can be seen using immersion oil and an ophthalmoscope set at 40 (green).
- Telangectasias can be found on the face, chest, lips, and mucus membranes.
- Decreased oral aperture and protrusion of the teeth are later clinical findings.
- Pulmonary examination may reveal fine rales in the bases if alveolitis is present.
- Cardiac auscultation can reveal irregular rhythms or a loud second heart sound with PHTN.

- Abdominal examination can show bloating with hyper- or hypoactive bowel sounds.
- Musculoskeletal examination may show tendon friction rubs and sclerodactaly.
- Proximal muscle strength may be diminished if myopathy is present.

DIFFERENTIAL DIAGNOSIS

The differential diagnosis of SSc involves other disorders with deposition of abnormal proteins into the skin: amyloidosis and scleromyxedema; inflammatory conditions: eosinophilic fasciitis, chronic graft-versus-host disease, sarcoidosis; and metabolic disorders: myxedema, porphyrias, and acromegaly. Once the SSc spectrum of disorders has been diagnosed, it is important to determine to which category the individual patient belongs (*Table 45*).

INVESTIGATIONS

The most important investigation is a good history and physical examination. Laboratory investigations include a CBC, chemistries, hepatic function testing, creatine kinase, and a urinalysis, looking for evidence of any organ involvement. Serologic testing is also very important. ANA is almost universally present. ANA subtypes are also commonly present and are mutually exclusive, which helps to predict disease activity (*Table 46*). Antitopoisomerase-1 (anti-SCL-70) is highly specific for diffuse SSc while the anticentromere antibody is very specific for the calcinosis, Raynaud's phenomenon, esophageal dysmotility, sclerodactyly, telangectasia (CREST) syndrome.

Additional diagnostic tests at baseline and for routine follow-up should be done to target commonly involved organs. These include a chest X-ray, pulmonary function testing (looking for restriction and diminished diffusing capacity), and a high-resolution CT examination to evaluate for ILD. A transthoracic echocardiogram and ECG should be performed to evaluate for PHTN and cardiac disease, and a right-heart catheterization may be required. Endoscopic evaluation, swallowing study, and manography may be needed to evaluate for GI problems.

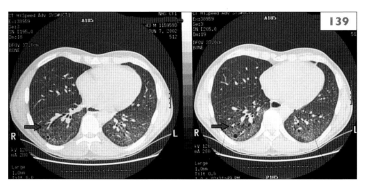

139 High resolution CT of the chest in a patient with diffuse scleroderma and pulmonary involvement, manifest by honeycombing and areas of ground glass appearance (arrows). (Courtesy of Dr GF Moore.)

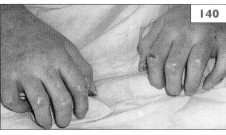

140 Hands of a patient with diffuse scleroderma with sclerodactyly, hide bound skin, digital flexion contractures, and areas of skin breakdown. (Courtesy of Dr GF Moore.)

Table 46 Autoantibodies in systemic sclerosis

Autoantibody (prevalence in disease)	Disease association	Clinical features
ANA (>95%)	Limited and diffuse SSc, CREST	
Antitopoisomerase 1 (Scl-70) (15–50%)	Diffuse SSc overlap	Skin thickening, ILD, tendon friction rubs
Anticentromere (15–20%)	CREST	Digital ischemia and amputation, PHTN
Anti-U1-RNP	Mixed connective tissue disease	ILD, PHTN, myositis
Anti-U3-RNP (fibrillarin) (8%)	Diffuse SSc	PHTN, myositis
Anti-RNA polymerase I/III (4–20%)	Diffuse SSc	Severe skin disease, renal crisis
Anti-PM/Scl (1–4%)	Limited SSc	Myositis

ANA: antinuclear antibody; CREST: calcinosis, Raynaud's phenomenon, esophageal dysmotility, sclerodactyly, telangiectasia; ILD: interstitial lung disease; PHTN: pulmonary hypertension; PM: polymyositis; RNA: ribonucleic acid; RNP: ribonucleoprotein; SSc: systemic sclerosis.

PROGNOSIS

Although no cure exists, current therapies have made a marked improvement in the morbidity and mortality of patients with SSc. Overall, prognosis depends on the organs involved, but the 5-year survival is now over 80%.

MANAGEMENT

Pharmacologic management should be targeted to the individual mechanism and organ system involved. Immunomodulatory drugs such as MTX, MMF, CTX, and AZA have all been used to control the inflammatory features of SSc such as skin disease and ILD, although evidence for their use is lacking. GCs are also used, but cautiously. There are no currently effective antifibrotic agents.

Vascular therapies are used to prevent vasospasm. These include calcium channel blockers and phosphodiesterase inhibitors. Additional agents are prostacyclins, endothelin receptor blockers, and angiotensin II receptor blockers. Sympathectomy is occasionally required to control severe RP. PHTN is usually treated in conjunction with a pulmonologist. SSc renal crisis is treated with ACE inhibitors, as it is a high renin state. Aspirin and statin drugs are also employed to mediate vascular endothelial damage. SSc patients with gastroesophageal reflux should receive proton pump inhibitors (PPIs).

Mixed connective tissue disease and undifferentiated connective tissue disease

DEFINITION

Mixed connective tissue disease (MCTD) is a clinical syndrome characterized by the presence of high titer, anti-RNP autoantibody and a combination of manifestations seen in several autoimmune diseases to include SLE, SSc, and polymyositis (PM).

Undifferentiated CTD (UCTD) is said to be present when the patient has features of an autoimmune disease, primarily in the SLE family, but does not meet diagnostic criteria for a specific recognizable clinical syndrome. Overlap syndromes occur when patients satisfy diagnostic criteria for more than one definable autoimmune disease, such as the combination of RA and SLE (so-called 'rhupus').

EPIDEMIOLOGY AND ETIOLOGY

There is a paucity of epidemiology data on MCTD with an etiology that remains poorly defined. The prevalence of MCTD is felt to be less than SLE and RA but greater than PM and SSc. There are no apparent racial or ethnic variations in disease incidence. The average age of onset is 37 years of age with a range of 5–80 years old. Like many other autoimmune diseases, MCTD is more common in females in a ratio similar to SLE (10:1). By definition, the epidemiology and etiology of UCTD are not well defined.

PATHOGENESIS

As with many other autoimmune diseases, genetic and environmental factors are important in the pathogenesis of MCTD. Immune dysregulation, with involvement of both B cells and T cells along with their cytokines, is important for disease onset. The importance of B cells is confirmed by the presence of autoantibodies targeting ribonucleoprotein (RNP). Though anti-RNP antibody positivity is necessary for the diagnosis, they have not been proven to be pathogenic. T cells also appear to play a central role in the pathogenesis of MCTD by producing pro-inflammatory cytokines leading to cellular recruitment important in the propagation of cellular and tissue inflammation. There is also evidence of the importance of the apoptotically modified self antigen.

CLINICAL HISTORY AND PHYSICAL EXAMINATION

The primary clinical features of MCTD are RP (**141**), hand and finger swelling, arthralgias, esophageal involvement (dysmotility and gastro-esophageal reflux), myopathy, and pulmonary manifestations which occur concurrently or sequentially (*Table 47*). The most frequent 'lupus-like' manifestation is arthralgia or nondeforming polyarthritis. Severe skin changes (e.g. sclero-dactyly) are more characteristic of PSS. In contrast to SLE, MCTD is only rarely characterized by renal involvement. Mild myositis with normal EMG are the most common muscle finding in MCTD, though there are cases of more severe involvement.

Pulmonary involvement can be severe in MCTD and is the most common disease-related source of mortality. Patients may have pleuritis, cough, dyspnea, or other physical findings of ILD, or PHTN.

Esophogeal dysmotility, similar to that observed in SSc, with its related symptoms, is common in MCTD. Most patients will have relatively mild symptoms with dysphagia being less common. Less common GI manifestations include pseudodiverticulum, bacterial overgrowth, and malabsorption, again similar to SSc.

Patients with UCTD may have a multitude of complaints, but will not have a definable, systemic, autoimmune disease. A typical patient may be a young female with joint pain, fatigue, and a positive ANA. In this scenario, the clinician may suspect a yet undiagnosed SLE patient or a patient in transition toward 'full blown lupus'.

Sjögren's syndrome (SS) SS is the most common overlap diagnosis and can be seen with RA, SLE, PM, SSc, and MCTD. These patients may have typical findings of SS syndrome described in the SS syndrome section.

DIFFERENTIAL DIAGNOSIS

Since MCTD has features of many autoimmune diseases, the differential includes these diagnoses. The astute clinician will realize that the presence of an anti-RNP in the correct clinical setting is consistent with MCTD. As with other auto-immune disease patients, one must always be diligent to exclude infection, especially in immunosuppressed patients.

Table 47 Frequency of clinical features in mixed connective tissue disease

Clinical feature	Present at onset (%)
Raynaud's phenomenon	90
Joint symptoms	90
Swollen hands	65
Esophageal disease	50
Pulmonary symptoms	45
Sclerodactyly	35
Serositis	35
Skin rash	30
Myositis	35
Hepatomegaly/splenomegaly	20
Renal disease	5
Neurological disease	<5

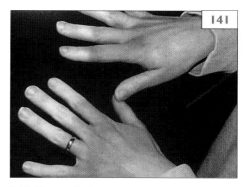

141 Raynaud's phenomenon in a young patient with mixed connective tissue disease manifest by high-titer antinuclear antibody and antiribonucleoprotein antibody; note the well-demarcated palor in multiple digits of both hands. (Courtesy of Dr GF Moore.)

INVESTIGATIONS

MCTD is characterized by a positive ANA and a positive anti-RNP antibody (RNP is an extractable antigen and belongs to a group of small nuclear ribonucleoproteins). In MCTD, the anti-RNP is the only specific ANA present. Other laboratory features may be common but are nonspecific and may be seen in other autoimmune diseases (*Table 48*).

Because pulmonary complications are common and lead to significant morbidity and mortality, routine pulmonary function testing and echocardiogram to screen for evidence of PHTN should be considered. If PHTN is suspected based on pulmonary function testing or echocardiogram findings, right-heart catheterization should be undertaken to confirm the presence of PHTN and rule out secondary causes such as chronic thromboembolic disease. A high-resolution chest CT is indicated if there is a suspicion of interstitial lung disease.

HISTOLOGY

Autopsy studies have shown proliferative vascular lesions which are often widespread. Plasmacyte-containing inflammation and vasculitis have also been reported. In patients with significant pulmonary involvement, pathology may demonstrate interstitial fibrosing pneumonitis or alveolitis, obliterative vasculopathy with intimal proliferation, and medial hypertrophy with minimal vasculitis.

PROGNOSIS

There is a low incidence of life-threatening renal disease and neurological disease in MCTD. The major mortality risk is from pulmonary complications, particularly the presence of PHTN. In general, patients with MCTD have a better prognosis than SLE or SSc.

Patients with UCTD tend to have a relatively benign disease course compared to patients with definable CTD. Individuals with overlap syndromes will have a prognosis dependent on the overlapping disease entities involved.

MANAGEMENT

The treatment of MCTD is guided by the manifestation that is being managed. Arthritis and serositis are treated with NSAIDs and possibly low-dose prednisone. Antimalarials (e.g. HCQ) may have a steroid-sparing effect and may have a role in mild to moderate disease, particularly with

Table 48 Laboratory findings in mixed connective tissue disease

Laboratory finding	Frequency (%)
Antinuclear antibody	100
Antiribonucleoprotein antibody	100
Anemia	75
Leukopenia	75
Rheumatoid factor	50

articular manifestations. As with other systemic autoimmune diseases, end-organ involvement, myositis, or life-threatening disease manifestations are frequently treated with immunomodulating agents such as AZA, CTX, and MTX, often in combination with higher-dose GCs. Adjuvant therapies may also be important for other specific disease manifestations:

- Calcium channel blockers for RP.
- Vasodilators for PHTN.
- PPIs for severe esophageal reflux.

Relapsing polychondritis

DEFINITION
Relapsing polychondritis (RPC) is a rare, episodic, progressive, and often destructive condition of presumed autoimmune etiology which manifests as recurrent inflammation of cartilaginous tissues.

EPIDEMIOLOGY AND ETIOLOGY
RPC is a rare disease with incidence of approximately 3.5/100 000. The mean age of diagnosis for RPC is in the 40s and 50s; however, it has been reported in individuals ranging from 6 to 87 years of age. RPC is more common in Caucasians than those of other ethnicities and has an approximately equal gender distribution. Approximately one-third of cases occur in association with another condition, most notably systemic vasculitis and myelodysplastic syndrome. The etiology of RPC is unknown, although genetic predisposition appears to play a role given reported associations with the presence of HLA-DR4 alleles (MHC class II).

PATHOGENESIS
The pathogenesis of RPC remains poorly defined. Antibodies to collagen (type II, IX, and XI) are observed in RPC and may play a role in disease pathogenesis.

CLINICAL HISTORY AND PHYSICAL EXAMINATION
RPC has abrupt and variable presentation with constitutional symptoms (fatigue, weight loss, fever, lymphadenopathy, and liver enlargement) common. Two sets of diagnostic criteria for RPC have been proposed: 1) the McAdam criteria (*Table 49*) require a compatible biopsy in addition to clinical features; and 2) the Michet criteria (*Table 50*), which do not require biopsy confirmation. Signs and symptoms of RPC are dependent on the tissues involved:
- Auricular/hearing (**142**): Most common presenting sign, most often bilateral (pain, swelling, warmth, and red/purple discoloration of the ear, sparing earlobe); it has a relapsing–remitting pattern and may leave a floppy pina or 'cauliflower deformity;' conductive loss occurs due to stenosis of the external auditory canal or Eustachian tube; sensorineural loss (± vestibular dysfunction) is due to vasculitis.

Table 49 Diagnostic criteria for relapsing polychondritis (McAdam, 1976)

Presence of three or more of the following:

Bilateral auricular chondritis

Nonerosive, seronegative inflammatory arthritis

Nasal chondritis

Ocular inflammation

Respiratory tract chondritis

Audio-vestibular damage

Table 50 Diagnostic criteria for relapsing polychondritis (Michet, 1986)

Major criteria

Proven inflammatory episodes involving auricular cartilage

Proven inflammatory episodes involving nasal cartilage

Proven inflammatory episodes involving laryngotracheal cartilage

Minor criteria or

Ocular inflammation (conjunctivitis, keratitis, episcleritis, uveitis)

Hearing loss

Vestibular dysfunction

Seronegative inflammatory arthritis

Diagnosis is made by two major criteria or one major plus two minor criteria; histological examination of affected cartilage is not required.

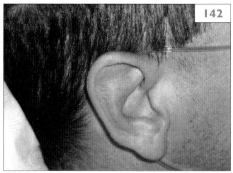

142 Auricular chondritis; erythema of the external ear with relative sparing of the ear lobe. (Courtesy of Dr GF Moore.)

- Ocular (**143**): Most common effect is episcleritis or scleritis.
- Nasal (**144**): Distal nasal septum is affected with progression to a saddle nose deformity possible.
- Airway: Dyspnea, cough, stridor, and hoarseness are common; tracheomalacia is the most common cause of airway symptoms; laryngotracheal chondritis occurs in ~50% and may manifest as anterior neck pain (over the thyroid cartilage); other symptoms include vocal cord palsy; subglottic or bronchial stenosis; inspiratory obstruction; tracheal and bronchial stenosis; bronchiectasis; and costochondritis.
- Cardiac: Late manifestation; aortic regurgitation is the most common symptom; others include mitral regurgitation; myocarditis; pericarditis; and conduction system defects.
- Arthritis/arthralgias: Frequent presenting symptom (70%); there is predilection for MCPs, PIPs, knees, ankles, wrists, metatarsal–phalangeal joints [MTPs], elbows, cervical, and/or lumbar spine; intermittent, migratory, nonerosive.
- Vasculitis: Medium/large vessel distribution.
- Renal: Microhematuria, proteinuria, or an abnormal kidney biopsy; poor prognosis; may be due to overlapping vasculitis; there is association with arthritis.
- Dermatologic: Oral aphthous ulcers; leukoclastic vasculitis.
- Neurologic: Cranial nerve involvement; central and peripheral nervous system involvement are uncommon; may be secondary to vasculitis.

DIFFERENTIAL DIAGNOSIS
The differential diagnosis of RPC is very broad and includes infections such as necrotizing otitis externa from *Pseudomonas aeurginosa*, tuberculosis, syphilis, leprosy, cellulitis, leishmaniasis, or acute sinusitis. Notably, infection of the ear does not spare the ear lobe as is seen in RPC. Other autoimmune diseases must be considered such as systemic vasculitis, RA, and spondyloarthropathies. Trauma, frostbite, tumors, amyloidosis, sarcoidosis, asthma/chronic bronchitis, Marfan syndrome, Ehlers–Danlos syndrome, medial cystic necrosis, tracheobronchopathia osteochondroplastica, and rhinoscleroma also need to be ruled out.

INVESTIGATIONS
Tissue biopsy of the involved pinna should be performed during an acute flare (see Histology). Nonspecific inflammatory markers may be useful to monitor disease activity; however, there are no laboratory tests specific for RPC. ANA is characteristically negative. ANCA (both MPO and PR3 specificity) have been observed. Antibodies to martrilin-1, cartilage oligometric matrix protein (COMP), collagen-type II, collagen-type IX, and collagen-type XI may be seen in RPC; however, none are sensitive and specific enough to be routinely useful in diagnosis.

Patients with RPC should be screened with pulmonary function testing (PFTs), ECG, chest X-ray, and transthoracic echocardiogram at baseline and over follow-up, as needed. Flow-volume loops are helpful in the assessment of possible intra- or extrathoracic pulmonary obstruction (**145**). Patients with murmur or unexplained dyspnea should undergo PFTs, ECG, and echocardiogram. If PFTs are abnormal or respiratory symptoms are unexplained, chest CT or MRI should be performed to evaluate for thickening of the soft tissues lining the larynx, trachea, and bronchi, collapse of the lumen, and/or calcification of the airways. CT, magnetic resonance angiography, ultrasound, and conventional angiography may be used to evaluate for aneurysms, vasculitis, or thrombosis. Bronchoscopy should not be done routinely due to risk of respiratory decomposition.

Joint aspiration in RPC-related arthritis demonstrates a noninflammatory synovial fluid, and joint radiography is typically normal without erosions.

HISTOLOGY
Tissue biopsy suggestive of RPC shows cartilage with degenerative changes and the presence of an inflammatory infiltrate which invades the cartilage from the periphery inward with neutrophils, lymphocytes, and plasma cells. Immunofluorescence may show the presence of Ig and complement.

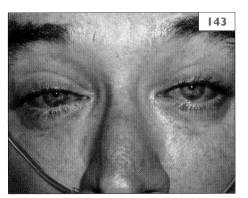

143 Episcleritis in a patient with relapsing polychondritis. (Courtesy of Dr GF Moore.)

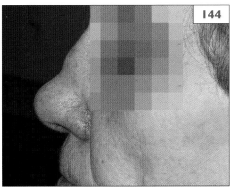

144 Saddle nose deformity caused by nasal chondritis. (Courtesy of Dr GF Moore.)

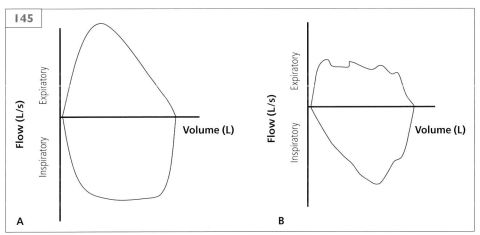

145 Representations of normal flow volume loop **(A)** and flow volume loop from patient with relapsing polychondritis with tracheomalacia and variable intrathoracic obstruction **(B)**.

PROGNOSIS

RPC has a generally favorable prognosis with 8-year survival reported to exceed 90%. The most common cause of death is from pulmonary involvement with both airway collapse and infection, followed by cardiac involvement. Systemic vasculitis and renal failure also increase mortality in patients with RPC.

MANAGEMENT

There are no prospective, randomized, controlled studies on which to base treatment; however, prednisone 10–20 mg/day is traditionally used for mild to moderate auricular and nasal chondritis or arthritis. For sensorineural hearing loss, vestibular symptoms, ocular involvement, respiratory compromise, vascular and renal complications, 1 mg/kg/day of prednisone or its equivalent is recommended. Topical steroid therapy is not effective for ocular manifestations. GCs may decrease the frequency, duration, and severity of flares, but do not stop disease progression. NSAIDs and colchicine may be useful for arthralgias/arthritis. Case reports of numerous immune modulating therapies (e.g. CTX, MTX) exist; however, none have proven superiority.

In acute flares with airway involvement, nebulized, racemic epinephrine may be useful. Tracheotomy may be required in severe, localized, subglottic involvement. Bronchial stenting to maintain airway patency has been used in select circumstances. Cardiac valve replacement may be required; however, it carries high short-term mortality rates with complications attributed to persistent inflammation and GC therapy. If cardiac valve replacement must be performed, prophylactic complete replacement of the ascending aorta with a graft that includes the aortic valve in patients with severe aortic insufficiency has been shown to limit postoperative complications.

Vasculitis

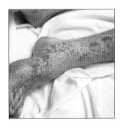
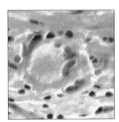
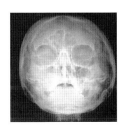
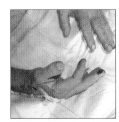

Introduction

DEFINITION

Vasculitis refers to a clinically heterogeneous group of disorders characterized by inflammation of blood vessels. Depending on the disorder, vasculitis may affect vessels of all sizes, including both arteries and veins. Vascular inflammation (primarily related to leukocyte migration and infiltration) leads to luminal narrowing of blood vessels resulting in clinical manifestations secondary to ischemic injury.

PATHOGENESIS

Vasculitis is most often classified according to the size of the primary blood vessels involved, recognizing that some forms of vasculitis can simultaneously affect arteries and veins of varying size (*Table 51*). At one extreme, large-vessel vasculitides are characterized by involvement of the aorta (aortitis) and its major branches, while at the other extreme, small-vessel vasculitides have their primary manifestation in the skin where small arterioles and capillaries are abundant.

Other classifications in vasculitis are based on characteristic laboratory findings (antinuclear antibody [ANA] or antineutrophil cytoplasmic antibody [ANCA]), the identification of other known triggers (most often microbial pathogens), or entities related to an underlying rheumatic condition. Examples of these classifications include:

- ANCA-associated vasculitis (e.g. Wegener's granulomatosis, Churg–Strauss syndrome, microscopic polyangiitis).
- Rheumatoid vasculitis seen as a complication of rheumatoid arthritis (RA).

Table 51 Classification of vasculitis based on vessel size involved

Small-vessel

Drug-induced (hypersensitivity)
Connective tissue diseases (SLE, Sjögren's)
Infections (HCV, HIV) and cryoglobulinemia
Malignancy-associated (lymphoproliferative diseases)
Urticarial vasculitis
Henoch–Schönlein purpura (**146**)

Medium-vessel

Polyarteritis nodosa (**147**)

Mixed small- and medium-vessel

Rheumatoid arthritis
Systemic lupus erythematosus
Microscopic polyangitis
Wegener's granulomatosis (**148**)
Churg–Strauss syndrome

Large-vessel

Giant cell arteritis
Takayasu arteritis (**149**)

HCV: hepatitis C virus; HIV: human immunodeficiency virus; SLE: systemic lupus erythematosus.

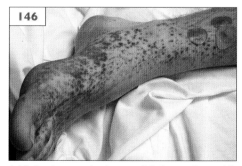

146 Leukocytoclastic vasculitis in a patient with Henoch–Schönlein purpura.

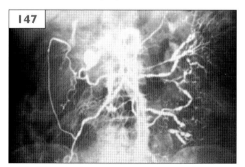

147 Abnormal mesenteric angiogram from a patient with polyarteritis nodosa.

- Lupus-related vasculitis seen as a complication of systemic lupus erythematosus (SLE).
- Infection-related vasculitis: infections known to be associated with vasculitis include but are not limited to:
  - Syphilis (aortitis).
  - Hepatitis C (HCV) (mixed cryoglobulinemia, MC).
  - Hepatitis B (HBV) (polyarteritis nodosa, PAN).
  - Human immunodeficiency virus (HIV) (MC).
  - Salmonella (tropic for atheromatous plaques).

In evaluating a patient with suspected idiopathic vasculitis, consideration must be given to the noninflammatory conditions that may closely mimic vasculitis (*Table 52*).

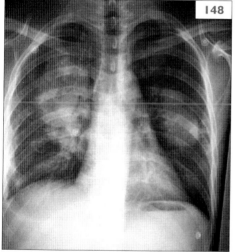

148 Pulmonary opacities in a patient with Wegener's granulomatosis.

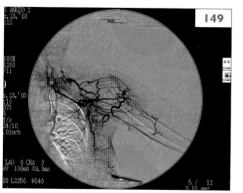

149 Abnormal upper extremity angiogram in a patient with Takayasu's arteritis.

Table 52 Mimics of vasculitis (adapted from Molloy & Langford, *Current Opinion in Rheumatology* 2008;20:29–34)

CNS vasculitis

Other rheumatic diseases (sarcoidosis, Behçet's)
Infection
Malignancy
Cerebral vasospasm
Atherosclerosis
Fibromuscular dysplasia
Thromboembolic disease
Moya-Moya and arteriovenous malformation
Leukoencephalopathy including progressive multifocal leukoencephalopathy and reversible posterior leukoencephalopathy

Small- and medium-vessel

Viral infections (HCV, HBV)
Endocarditis, sepsis
Atherosclerosis
Malignancy
Hereditary disorders (Ehler–Danlos)
Fibromuscular dysplasia
Thromboembolic disease
Midline granuloma and illicit drug use (cocaine may cause necrotizing upper airway inflammation closely mimicking Wegener's)

Large-vessel

Infections (e.g. endocarditis)
Atherosclerosis
Hereditary disorders (Marfan's, Ehler–Danlos)
Fibromuscular dysplasia
Inflammatory aortic aneurysm/retroperitoneal fibrosis

HBV: hepatitis B virus; HCV: hepatitis C virus.

CLINICAL HISTORY AND PHYSICAL EXAMINATION

The clinical manifestations of vasculitis vary based on the underlying disease entity, recognizing the substantial overlap in signs and symptoms across different vasculitides. Common signs and symptoms by organ system are shown in *Table 53*.

INVESTIGATIONS

A targeted evaluation is based on the presenting signs and symptoms. Vasculitis should be suspected in any rapidly evolving multisystem illness, particularly those characterized by an inflammatory pathology.

Laboratory tests that may be helpful in the evaluation of a patient with suspected vasculitis include:

- Erythrocyte sedimentation rate (ESR) and C-reactive protein (CRP): almost universally elevated in systemic vasculitis and can be tracked with treatment response.
- Complete blood count (CBC – leukocytosis, eosinophilia in select cases).
- Creatinine and urinalysis (UA) to examine kidney function.
- Serum chemistries, including liver function tests.
- Serologies including ANCA, ANA, rheumatoid factor (RF), complements (C3, C4), and cryoglobulins.
- Serologies for hepatitis B/C and HIV.

Select imaging tests may also be helpful and are discussed under each specific disease entity. These may include plain radiography and advanced imaging techniques including magnetic resonance imaging (MRI), computed tomography (CT), and angiography.

The diagnosis of vasculitis often requires a tissue biopsy with the common biopsy sites including the skin, lung, kidney, nerve (most commonly the sural nerve), sinuses, and less often, the brain.

MANAGEMENT

Treatments of specific forms of vasculitis are discussed in the following sections. In general, effective treatment strategies are based on the following principles:

- Eliminating or treating any identifiable trigger or underlying cause.
- The judicious use of anti-inflammatory agents, often including combinations of glucocorticoids (GCs), alkylating agents (cyclophosphamide, CTX), or other immunomodulating drugs.

Table 53 Common signs and symptoms of vasculitis

Constitutional
Fevers, weight loss, anorexia

Musculoskeletal
Arthralgias/arthritis
Myalgias/myositis

Skin
Purpura
Digital ischemia/necrosis and pain
Livedo reticularis

Gastrointestinal
Abdominal pain
Hematochezia

Eye
Vision loss

Renal
Hematuria, manifestations secondary to azotemia

Cardiovascular
Limb claudication
Chest pain
Hypertension

Pulmonary and upper airway
Dyspnea
Hemoptysis, nose bleeds
Chronic sinusitis/otitis
Hearing loss

Neurological
Mental status change/confusion
Headache
Cerebrovascular accident
Polyneuropathy or mononeuritis multiplex

Giant cell arteritis and polymyalgia rheumatica

DEFINITION
Giant cell arteritis (GCA), sometimes referred to as temporal arteritis, is a systemic vasculitis affecting the large and medium vessels of the proximal aorta, classically involving the extracranial branches of the carotid artery. Polymyalgia rheumatica (PMR) is a systemic, inflammatory disorder in which patients present with painful stiffness of the shoulders, neck, and pelvic girdle. GCA and PMR are closely associated conditions, occurring concomitantly in many patients.

EPIDEMIOLOGY AND ETIOLOGY
GCA constitutes the most common form of systemic vasculitis in adults. The incidence of GCA is dependent upon age, race, and ethnic background, with patients of northern European descent at highest risk. Patients of southern European, Asian, and African-American descent are at much lower risk of developing GCA. The incidence of GCA reaches 20–30 per 100 000 persons aged 50 years and older. GCA affects females two to three times more commonly than males.

PMR is a common illness with an incidence rate of approximately 50 per 100 000 persons aged 50 years and older. PMR shares many epidemiologic characteristics with GCA, including age and ethnic background, and is commonly seen in patients with biopsy-proven GCA.

It is estimated that approximately 15–20% of patients with PMR have concomitant GCA and that approximately 50–70% of patients with GCA suffer from concomitant PMR. The cause(s) of GCA and/or PMR have yet to be fully elucidated. Genetic and environmental risk factors likely play a role, based on the geographic distribution and seasonal variation seen in both diseases.

PATHOGENESIS
Recent work has shed light on the pathogenesis of GCA, and demonstrates the important role dendritic cells play in the initiation of vasculitis. Immature dendritic cells function as antigen-presenting cells at the media–adventia border in normal arteries. In GCA, dendritic cells are activated to produce cytokines and other co-stimulatory signals which recruit and activate CD4+ T cells and macrophages in the vessel wall.

Activated T cells and macrophages release numerous cytokines including interferon (IFN)-γ, interleukin (IL)-1, IL-2, IL-6, transforming growth factor (TGF)-β, and nitric oxide. Together these cytokines are responsible for the intimal thickening, angioneogenesis, and formation of giant cells within the arterial wall. GCA is classically associated with giant cells, although these are seen in only 50% of biopsies.

Patients with PMR exhibit high levels of IL-1 and IL-6, providing evidence of activated macrophages and dendritic cells; however, these patients do not exhibit T cell-mediated IFN-γ production. This lack of IFN-γ explains the paucity of arterial inflammation seen in PMR when compared to GCA. The inflammatory response seen with PMR may provide protection from the ischemic complications of GCA through increased IL-6-induced angiogenesis.

CLINICAL HISTORY AND PHYSICAL EXAMINATION
Clinical features of GCA include:
- Headache: The most common symptom (~75%); temporal/occipital distribution; scalp tenderness; headaches can be nocturnal.
- Visual loss: Affects ~20%; due to narrowing/occlusion of the posterior ciliary artery leading to optic neuropathy resulting in transient/permanent visual loss; it is usually unilateral at onset with contralateral eye involvement more common if untreated; diplopia occurs due to ischemia in extraocular muscles; formal ophthalmologic examination is essential in patients with visual symptoms.
- Jaw or tongue claudication: <40%, highly specific for GCA.
- Scalp tenderness.
- Constitutional symptoms and symptoms of overlapping PMR: Fever, malaise, weight loss, or depression; fevers are typically low grade, but high fevers are not uncommon and may be the only symptom; GCA is a common cause of fever of unknown origin in older adults.
- Other: Include cough, sore throat, transient ischemia attack (TIA), stroke, neuropathies, or a myriad of other atypical symptoms; such symptoms should be included in the differential diagnosis of atypical head and neck symptoms in the elderly.

Clinical features of PMR include:

- Pain over the shoulder, neck, hips, or pelvis: New onset bilateral shoulder pain in an elderly patient should raise suspicion of PMR (muscle strength is typically normal on examination); pain may be nocturnal and exacerbated with activity.
- Morning stiffness.
- Constitutional symptoms.
- Pain, tenderness, swelling (synovitis) in peripheral joints; may closely mimic RA.

DIFFERENTIAL DIAGNOSIS

Small- or medium-vessel vasculidities including Wegener's granulomatosis or polyarteritis nodosa (PAN), amyloidosis, lymphoma, atypical infections, and atherosclerotic disease should all be included in the differential diagnosis of GCA. PMR may mimic many diseases and must be differentiated from early RA, neoplasm, polymyositis, bacterial endocarditis, and remitting, seronegative synovitis with pitting edema (RS$_3$PE) (**150**).

INVESTIGATIONS

Giant cell arteritis

The definitive diagnosis of GCA is based on temporal artery biopsy. The sensitivity and specificity of temporal artery biopsy approaches 95% at experienced centers. If possible, a 2–3 cm section of temporal artery should be removed to evaluate adequately, as GCA often produces 'skip lesions' that may be missed. Biopsy is well-tolerated with low morbidity if done by experienced surgeons. Unilateral biopsy is often sufficient; however, in cases with a high likelihood of GCA and a negative biopsy, a second biopsy should be obtained. Many experts recommend bilateral biopsies initially, as this may provide the diagnosis in up to 13% of patients with negative unilateral biopsies.

The timing of the biopsy is important and all attempts should be made to obtain tissue within 1–2 weeks of initiating treatment; however, biopsies may remain positive for months after initiation of GCs in some patients. In patients with a high probability of GCA, the timing of the biopsy should not interfere with the initiation of GCs, as blindness can occur early in the disease, prior to steroid initiation.

In GCA, similar to PMR, patients often have elevated inflammatory markers, normocytic anemia, and elevated liver function tests. Up to 10% of patients with GCA will have an ESR below 50 mm/hr, but nearly all will have elevated levels of CRP. IL-6 is often elevated in patients with PMR and GCA, although commercial testing for this cytokine is not widely available at this time.

Imaging may play an important role in the diagnosis of some patients with GCA, especially in those with large-vessel involvement and sparing of the temporal artery. Ultrasound may show a 'hypoechoic halo effect' around the temporal artery prior to initiation of GCs. In addition, MRI and MR angiography may show temporal artery inflammatory changes consistent with GCA, and have the benefit of evaluating the more proximal large vessels near the aorta (**151, 152**). At the present time, both imaging modalities lack the sensitivity to replace biopsy.

Polymyalgia rheumatica

The diagnosis of PMR is based on clinical history and examination, elevated inflammatory markers, and response to GCs. Most patients with PMR have ESRs of greater than 40 mm/hr, but a normal ESR does not exclude PMR. CRP is highly sensitive for the diagnosis of patients with PMR, and is especially helpful in patients with a low or normal ESR. Patients with PMR may also exhibit elevated alkaline phosphatase levels, and commonly present with a normocytic, normochromic anemia.

Radiographic evidence of PMR can be seen with numerous modalities including MRI and ultrasound, although in most patients the diagnosis of PMR is evident without radiographic testing. MRI and ultrasound are both highly sensitive for PMR, often demonstrating synovitis or inflammatory bursitis (particularly subacromial bursitis in patients with shoulder pain). MRI and ultrasound may be most helpful in patients with atypical symptoms or clinical response.

HISTOLOGY

Biopsy of the temporal artery classically reveals inflammatory infiltrates of the intima and muscularis while the internal elastic lamina is often disrupted and frayed. Multinucleated giant cells

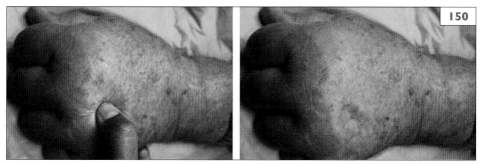

150 Pitting edema of the hand of a patient with remitting seronegative synovitis with pitting edema, a condition that frequently overlaps and may be confused with polymyalgia rheumatica (PMR). The marked peripheral edema shown would be uncommon in PMR. (Reprinted with permission, Quadrant HealthCom, NJ; Bucaloiu et al., Remitting seronegative symmetrical synovitis with pitting edema syndrome in a rural tertiary care practice: a retrospective analysis. *Mayo Clinical Proceedings* 2007;**82**(12):1510–5.)

151, 152 Angiograms in a patient with biopsy-proven GCA with diffuse large artery involvement. **151**: Near complete occlusion of right subclavian artery (arrow); **152**: near complete occlusion of left femoral artery (arrowhead) and tapering of right femoral artery (large arrow).

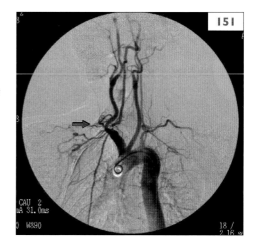

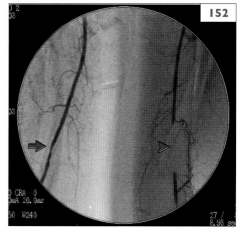

may also be seen (although are not essential) (**153–155**). Although biopsy is rarely indicated in PMR, histology of involved synovium may show infiltrates characteristic of an inflammatory arthritis.

PROGNOSIS

The prognosis of patients with PMR is usually good, with most adverse effects related to concurrent GCA and the use of corticosteroids. GCA prognosis is related to early initiation of corticosteroids to prevent blindness, long-term morbidity due to corticosteroids, and its propensity to induce aneurysm years after diagnosis. Patients with GCA are at 17 times greater risk of developing thoracic aneurysm and 2.4 times greater risk of developing abdominal aneurysm when compared with their peers. Evidence-based guidelines regarding the optimal screening tool(s) are lacking, but experts recommend yearly screening in all patients without significant risk factors for adverse surgical outcomes.

MANAGEMENT
Giant cell arteritis

The treatment of GCA is based upon high-dose GCs to avoid the potential ocular manifestations of the disease. Steroids are highly effective agents in the treatment of GCA, despite a toxic side-effect profile and increased morbidity. Patients with suspected GCA should be started on 40–60 mg of prednisone equivalent. In patients with loss of vision, there is limited evidence that higher doses of steroids reverse the ocular damage; thus, many clinicians recommend high-dose pulse therapy to preserve vision in the unaffected eye. Approximately 80–90% of patients with GCA will suffer GC side-effects, with nearly 50% suffering two or more adverse events. The tapering approach and use of steroid-sparing agents in the treatment of GCA is similar to that used in PMR (see below). Prednisone dose should be tapered by approximately 10% after 3–4 weeks, and slowly thereafter every few weeks to months, with a goal of 5–10 mg prednisone equivalent per day by 9 months. Tapering schedules should be guided by symptoms and by monitoring of acute phase responses. Many patients will experience minor flares, and the dose should be increased by 5–10 mg. A tapering schedule involving steroids every other day is ineffective, and should not be used.

In addition to corticosteroids, acetylsalicylic acid (aspirin, ASA) plays a vital role in the treatment of GCA. Studies have shown a significant reduction in the incidence of cranial ischemic events in patients on ASA therapy. A dose of 81–162 mg daily is sufficient and well tolerated by most patients.

Polymyalgia rheumatica

The management of PMR involves low-dose GCs, often for periods as long as 18–24 months. A dramatic and rapid response to steroids at doses of 10–20 mg daily (prednisone equivalent) is typical, making this a useful diagnostic tool in patients with suspected PMR. In patients without evidence of GCA who do not improve within the first week, many experts recommend increasing the dose of prednisone to 30 mg daily. If this fails to relieve symptoms, an alternative diagnosis should be sought. The patient should be maintained on 10–20 mg of prednisone daily for approximately 3–4 weeks, at which time tapering may begin if symptoms have resolved and inflammatory markers have normalized. Numerous tapering schedules have been proposed, with most slowly decreasing the dose of prednisone by 2.5 mg per month until the patient is on approximately 10 mg daily. At that time, a slower taper should be initiated with doses decreased by 1 mg every 6–8 weeks. PMR is commonly associated with flares, and many patients will develop toxicity from long-term corticosteroid use. Numerous steroid-sparing agents have been evaluated including methotrexate (MTX), azathioprine (AZA), and the antitumor necrosis factor (anti-TNF) agents, with conflicting results.

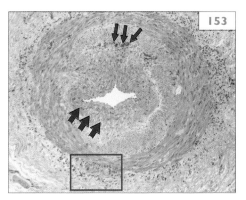

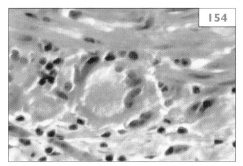

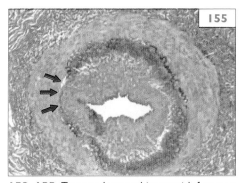

153–155 Temporal artery biopsy with features of healing GCA. **153**: Prominent intimal thickening including smooth muscle proliferation (bottom arrows) and neovascularization (upper arrows); rare adventitial, multinucleated giant cells are present (**153** inset and **154**). Alteration of internal elastic lamina with disruption (arrows, **155**) and reduplication is demonstrated on Verhoeff–Van Gieson elastin stain.

Takayasu's arteritis

DEFINITION

Takayasu's arteritis (TA) is an idiopathic, inflammatory disorder affecting the aorta and its major branches.

EPIDEMIOLOGY AND ETIOLOGY

TA most commonly affects women, with a female to male ratio of approximately 8:1. A majority of new cases of TA are diagnosed prior to age 40, but evidence is increasing that patients may develop TA into their fifth or sixth decade of life. The incidence varies worldwide, with Japan reporting an incidence of approximately 150 cases per million per year. In the US, the incidence falls to approximately two cases per million per year. Although numerous genetic and environmental causes have been investigated, etiologic risk factors for TA are not well understood.

PATHOGENESIS

TA shares striking pathologic similarities to GCA. Inflammatory cells, including T cells, dendritic cells, and macrophages are responsible for the inflammatory reaction leading to arterial stenosis, aneurysm, and occlusion.

CLINICAL HISTORY AND PHYSICAL EXAMINATION

TA commonly presents with symptoms of vascular stenosis, occlusion, or aneurysm. Early in the course of the disease, many patients experience nonspecific arthralgias, myalgias, and constitutional symptoms. Claudication of the upper and lower extremities is common with upper extremity involvement more commonly seen in early disease. Patients can develop cardiovascular complications including hypertension, congestive heart failure, myocardial ischemia, and valvular insufficiency, leading to increased morbidity and mortality. Central nervous system (CNS) manifestations may occur, and consist of TIAs, stroke, syncope, and visual changes. Complete loss of vision is much less common in TA when compared with GCA. In addition, TA may affect the skin, pulmonary arteries, and abdominal arteries.

Physical examination findings may include:
- Diminished peripheral pulses (TA has been called 'pulseless arteritis').
- Pallor and coolness of involved extremities.

- Blood pressure discrepancies with upper limb involvement (~50%).
- Audible arterial bruits over involved blood vessels (70% with carotid bruits).
- Aortic insufficiency murmur with proximal aortic involvement (~20%).

DIFFERENTIAL DIAGNOSIS

TA must be differentiated from other rheumatic causes of large vessel vasculitis (i.e. GCA, Behçet's disease), Ehlers–Danlos syndrome, infections, drug-induced vasculitis, atherosclerosis, and fibromuscular dysplasia (FMD). Diagnostic criteria for the diagnosis of TA are shown in *Table 54*.

INVESTIGATIONS

The diagnosis of TA is made primarily with imaging. Clinical signs of claudication, early cardiovascular disease, and unexplained constitutional symptoms should prompt early angiographic evaluation of the aorta and its branches (**156**). Inflammatory markers including ESR and CRP are typically elevated, but often lack significant correlation with disease progression. Angiographic evaluation may include conventional angiogram, CT angiography, or MR angiography. Ultrasonography and positron emission tomography (PET) imaging are less frequently used. Conventional contrast angiography may be beneficial in obtaining accurate measurement of central arterial pressures or allowing for therapeutic interventions, but is more invasive than other modalities in the diagnosis of TA. CT and MR angiography are highly sensitive and specific, and are considered the imaging modalities of choice for most cases of TA.

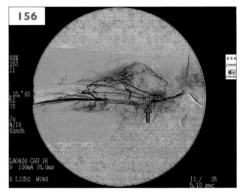

156 Arteriogram showing occlusion of the right subclavian artery (arrow) with marked collateralization in a patient with Takayasu's arteritis. (Courtesy of Dr GF Moore.)

Table 54 American College of Rheumatology criteria for the clinical diagnosis of Takayasu's arteritis (TA) (3 of 6 criteria needed for diagnosis)

Criterion	Definition
Age of onset <40 years	Development of symptoms or findings related to TA prior to the age of 40 years
Claudication of extremities	Development and worsening of fatigue and/or discomfort in muscles of one or more extremity while in use, especially in upper extremities
Decreased brachial artery pulse	Decreased pulsation of one or both brachial arteries
Blood pressure difference >10 mmHg	Difference of at least 10 mmHg in systolic blood pressure between arms
Bruit over subclavian arteries or aorta	Bruit audible on auscultation over one or both subclavian arteries or abdominal aorta
Arteriogram abnormality	Arteriographic narrowing or occlusion of the entire aorta, its primary branches, or large arteries in the proximal upper and lower extremities, not caused by atherosclerosis, fibromuscular dysplasia, or similar causes; changes are usually focal or segmental

HISTOLOGY

Given its primary involvement of large blood vessels, biopsy is rarely performed in TA. Histological examination of involved vessels shows similarities to findings in GCA. TA is characterized by panarteritis with T cell and dendritic cell infiltrates and smooth muscle proliferation. Multinucleated giant cells may also be present in TA. As in GCA, chronic disease may be characterized by progressive fibrosis.

PROGNOSIS

Most patients with TA exhibit a chronic disease but a small percentage of patients have self-limited disease. In patients with persistently active disease, mortality is estimated at 10–15% with a high percentage of excess deaths due to cardiac complications. Patients with TA also exhibit high levels of morbidity due to steroid-induced toxicity.

MANAGEMENT

TA is generally responsive to high-dose GCs. Daily doses of 60 mg of prednisone (or its equivalent) are usually effective in the treatment of active disease. However, TA is usually more difficult to treat than GCA with nearly all patients experiencing relapse or progression of disease with GC tapering. Small open studies evaluating the use of agents including MTX, AZA, and CTX have suggested a modest steroid-sparing effect when added to prednisone. None of these agents have been shown to be more effective than GCs in the treatment of TA.

In addition to medical therapy, surgical/invasive vascular interventions may be indicated in severe disease. Outcomes are best in patients with inactive disease undergoing bypass procedures, but angioplasty may have beneficial short-term effects. Most studies evaluating stents have been disappointing, and the placement of stents in TA should generally be avoided, particularly in the context of active inflammation.

ANCA-associated vasculitis – Wegener's granulomatosis, microscopic polyangiitis, and Churg–Strauss syndrome

DEFINITION

Three diseases, Wegener's granulomatosis (WG), microscopic polyangiitis (MPA), and Churg–Strauss syndrome (CSS), have shared pathologic, clinical, and laboratory features. Each of the diseases is a small- to medium-vessel inflammatory condition that is frequently (but not universally) characterized by a positive ANCA and multisystem involvement. The American College of Rheumatology has recently recommended that Wegener's granulomatosis be renamed 'granulomatosis with polyangitis'. Throughout this book the older, more conventional term of WG will be used.

EPIDEMIOLOGY AND ETIOLOGY

These diseases are uncommon with an incidence of approximately two per 100 000 people in the US. Each of the diseases is typically associated with a positive ANCA, but evidence for a precipitating event is not strong. Various etiologies have been proposed but remain unproven.

PATHOGENESIS

The presence of ANCA suggests an autoimmune response to unknown antigens that result in a small- to medium-vessel inflammatory response in the walls of the venules, capillaries and/or arterioles. ANCA presumably activates neutrophils which attack small blood vessels in the lungs, kidneys, and other affected tissues. Immunoglobulin or complement activation is not typically found (these conditions are often described as 'pauci-immune'). Glomerular disease manifested by focal necrosis, crescents, and minimal immunoglobulin deposition is demonstrated in most cases (particularly WG and MPA). Significant overlap between these diseases makes distinction between the different entities difficult at times.

CLINICAL HISTORY AND PHYSICAL EXAMINATION

WG and MPA can present with similar signs and symptoms. Upper airway symptoms include chronic sinusitis, nasal obstruction, saddle nose deformity, Eustachian and middle ear involvement, hearing loss (uncommon), as well as ophthalmic pain and visual disturbances. WG is a rare cause of proptosis resulting from an inflammatory pseudotumor of the orbit (**157a, b**). Epiglottal and tracheal involvement may result in hoarseness and signs of laryngeal obstruction. Pulmonary symptoms include hemoptysis, shortness of breath, and cough. Pulmonary examination may be completely normal or demonstrate wheezing (CSS). Rales and rhonchi may be found. Renal symptoms are usually absent but the patient may complain of hematuria, frequency, or foamy urine (related to underlying proteinuria). Late presentations include symptoms of uremia if the diagnosis is delayed. Rapid progression of symptoms may occur infrequently. Palpable purpura may be observed in all forms of ANCA-associated vasculitis (**158**). Arthralgias and frank arthritis may occasionally be present. Signs and symptoms of mononeuritis multiplex should be sought.

CSS often presents with asthma (classically adult-onset) with related symptoms of wheezing and dyspnea. Early in the disease course, symptoms are usually limited to the respiratory system. As the disease progresses, more systemic complaints/findings, such as mononeuritis multiplex, abdominal pain, and skin rashes including palpable purpura may become manifest.

DIFFERENTIAL DIAGNOSIS

Diffuse hemoptysis and hematuria should suggest one of the pulmonary–renal syndromes. In addition to WG and MPA, Goodpasture's syndrome and systemic lupus should be considered; the latter two diseases are typically ANCA negative. For patients with isolated upper respiratory involvement, other considerations include midline granuloma and illicit drug use (particularly cocaine).

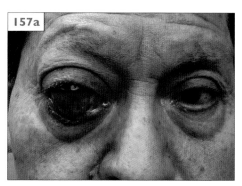

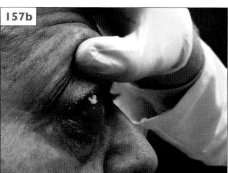

157a, b Wegener's granulomatosis has been recognized as a rare cause of proptosis (often unilateral), seen here in this 61-year-old presenting simultaneously with purpura, glomerlulonephritis, and cavitary lung lesions. (Courtesy of Dr GF Moore.)

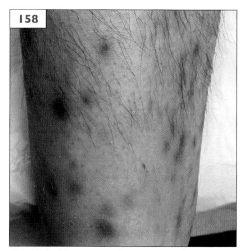

158 Palpable purpura (nonblanching) in a patient with Wegener's granulomatosis. (Courtesy of Dr GF Moore.)

INVESTIGATIONS

ANCA is a unique antibody associated with WG, MPA, and CSS. ANCA was originally described based on the pattern of immunofluorescence staining – cytoplasmic (C-ANCA) or perinuclear (P-ANCA). Cytoplasmic staining is more typical of WG while perinuclear staining is typical for MPA and CSS, the latter being relatively nonspecific. The antigens associated with cytoplasmic staining are proteinase 3 (PR3) and those associated with the perinuclear pattern are myeloperoxidase (MPO). Anti-PR3 and anti-MPO antibody testing are often performed as confirmatory tests. The utility of serial ANCA measurements to track treatment disease or predict disease relapse remains controversial.

Up to 90% of WG patients are ANCA positive (the PR3 antigen is responsible for the positive ANCA in over three-quarters of the patients). Up to 80% of MPA patients are ANCA positive. Both C-ANCA (and anti-PR3) and P-ANCA (anti-MPO) can be seen in MPA. CSS has a lower positivity for ANCA, usually in the range of 40–60% (MPO antigen).

Upper airway (sinuses and nasal passages), lower airway (lungs) and kidneys may be involved and should be evaluated. Sinus imaging studies (CT or radiograph, **159**) may show evidence of sinusitis. Radiographs of the chest may show nodular opacities, cavitary lesions and fleeting infiltrates but no specific finding is characteristic of the disease process (**160**).

CBC may show leukocytosis, thrombo-cytosis, and anemia of chronic disease related to systemic inflammation. Eosinophilia is characteristic of CSS. With renal involvement, proteinuria, hematuria, and red blood cell casts may be seen along with an elevated serum creatinine. Inflammatory markers including ESR and CRP are almost universally elevated with active systemic disease and can be helpful in tracking treatment response. In contrast to forms of immune-complex mediated vasculitis, serum complements are usually normal in ANCA-associated vasculitis.

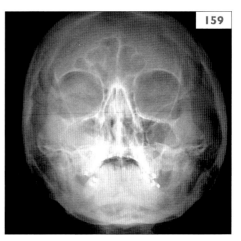

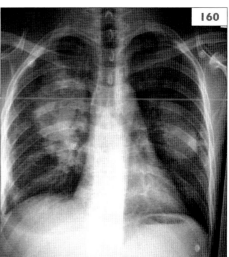

159, 160 Imaging studies from a patient with Wegener's granulomatosis. **159**: Sinus radiograph demonstrates opacification of the right maxillary sinus cavity; **160**: chest radiograph demonstrates bilateral nodular opacities. (Courtesy of Dr GF Moore.)

HISTOLOGY

Biopsy of involved tissues (kidney, lung, sinuses) is often critical in the evaluation of patients with suspected ANCA-associated vasculitis. All of the ANCA-associated diseases demonstrate a small- to medium-vessel inflammatory response in the walls of the venules, capillaries, and/or arterioles (**161**).

WG is characterized by necrotizing granulomatous inflammation affecting the upper airway, lungs, and kidneys. Giant cells are common findings. Crescentic glomerulonephritis is characteristic in renal pathology. MPA is similar to WG but does not typically form granulomas or have giant cells. CSS develops marked tissue eosinophilia and may have extravascular granulomas.

PROGNOSIS

When initially described, the prognosis in WG was typically fatal with an average survival of 5 months after diagnosis. The use of CTX has dramatically altered the prognosis with 75% of treated patients typically reaching remission and 87% surviving in the long term. Complications of CTX therapy are common. The titer of ANCA does not necessarily predict disease activity. A high serum creatinine (>5 mg/dl [>442 μmol/l]) is associated with poor renal survival and increased risk of end-stage renal disease and the need for chronic dialysis.

Large studies evaluating the prognosis for treatment in MPA and CSS are generally not available. Studies of MTX, AZA, mycophenolate, and leflunomide report remission rates of 35–74% in limited disease. Anti-TNF inhibition in addition to MTX and CTX may result in similar response rates when compared to placebo plus MTX and CTX, but may result in an increased incidence of solid cancers.

MANAGEMENT
Induction of remission

Standard management of WG, MPA, and CSS depends on the extent of the disease process and whether life-threatening complications are present. Studies in the literature primarily deal with response of WG to various treatment regimens. Severe organ involvement should be treated with CTX and high-dose corticosteroids. Corticosteroid therapy alone is inadequate. Oral daily CTX appears to have a small advantage over pulse intravenous CTX therapy, but has an increased incidence of side-effects (bone marrow suppression and hemorrhagic cystitis). Occasionally plasmapheresis is utilized. Studies with IV immunoglobulin (IVIG), anti-TNF drugs, rituximab, and other biologics have failed to show major improvement when compared with standard therapy.

Maintenance of remission

The early replacement of oral weekly MTX or daily AZA therapy for CTX may be effective for maintenance of remission and is usually associated with fewer drug-related complications. Treatment with trimethoprim sulfamethoxazole in WG localized to the upper airways may be beneficial.

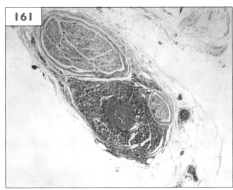

161 Sural nerve biopsy specimen from a patient with Churg–Strauss syndrome demonstrates inflammatory response in the walls of the vasa nervorum; note the marked luminal narrowing resulting in ischemia and nerve damage. (Courtesy of Dr GF Moore.)

Polyarteritis nodosa

DEFINITION

Polyarteritis nodosa (PAN) is a systemic vasculitis primarily affecting medium-sized muscular arteries. Though it typically spares veins and large arteries, it may occasionally involve small, muscular arteries. PAN has a predilection for the vasculature supplying the kidneys, gastrointestinal (GI) tract and the skin, though the lungs are almost universally spared.

EPIDEMIOLOGY AND ETIOLOGY

PAN has a slight male predominance (~2:1) and occurs in all ethnic groups. The peak age of onset is in the sixth decade though it may occur in all age groups. PAN is a rare form of vasculitis, with an incidence of fewer than 10 cases per million people annually, and comprises less than 5% of all systemic vasculitides. Most cases of PAN are idiopathic. Though it may occur in isolation, PAN is often associated with HBV infection and very rarely with hairy cell leukemia. In areas where the HBV vaccine is widely available, less than 10% of cases of PAN are associated with this virus. The clinical features of PAN are similar whether idiopathic or secondary to HBV infection.

PATHOGENESIS

Mechanisms involved in PAN-related vascular injury are not completely understood, but are thought to relate to immune complex formation. In the case of PAN secondary to HBV, the hepatitis surface antigen may act as the trigger for immune complex generation. In animal models of PAN, immune complexes activate the complement cascade, which leads to the infiltration of neutrophils. ANCAs do not appear to play a major role in the pathogenesis of PAN. It has been speculated that antiendothelial cell autoantibodies may also play a pathogenic role in PAN and other systemic vasculitides. The predominance of macrophages and cytotoxic T cells in biopsy specimens suggests that these inflammatory cells also play an important pathogenic role in PAN.

CLINICAL HISTORY AND PHYSICAL EXAMINATION

The symptoms of PAN usually present insidiously over weeks to months, though acute presentations have been described. Constitutional symptoms such as fever, weight-loss, malaise, and diffuse pain are common. Arthritis and arthralgias may be present and tend to be asymmetric, with large joint involvement. Virtually all symptoms in PAN are secondary to vascular ischemia. The kidneys are the most common organ involved in PAN but glomerular involvement is generally absent. Impaired renal function and hypertension often result from renal ischemia. Perinephric hematomas may result from ruptured aneurysms. New-onset hypertension in the setting of systemic symptoms should prompt an evaluation for PAN. Orchitis (generally unilateral) may manifest from ischemia of the testicular artery. GI manifestations are common and include diarrhea, nausea, vomiting, GI bleeding, and pain. Mesenteric ischemia due to involvement of the mesenteric vasculature supplying the small bowel may occur. Ischemia of the peripheral nerves may lead to mononeuritis multiplex.

Cutaneous manifestations are common and include palpable purpura, livedo reticularis, digital ischemia, splinter hemorrhages, ulcerations, and nodules. Coronary involvement is seldom clinically significant but aneurysms of the coronary vessels can be found. Other cardiac manifestations, such as congestive heart failure (secondary to hypertension), arrhythmias, and ischemia are less common.

DIFFERENTIAL DIAGNOSIS

The differential of PAN is broad and includes: ANCA-associated vasculitides, vasculitis secondary to connective tissue diseases (CTDs), cryoglobulinemia, thromboangiitis obliterans, FMD, segmental arteriolar mediolysis, radiation fibrosis, ergotism, syphilis, and vasculitis mimics (subacute bacterial endocarditis, embolic phenomena, hepatitides). Diagnostic criteria for PAN have been developed and are shown in *Table 55 Overleaf*.

INVESTIGATIONS

No tests are diagnostic; common abnormalities include: anemia, leukocytosis, elevated ESR and CRP; urinary sediment is generally bland, but mild hematuria and subnephrotic range proteinuria may be seen. Serologies including ANA and RF are generally absent; ANCAs also are generally negative though P-ANCA positivity with negative MPO/PR3 has been reported; serum complements (C3, C4) are generally normal.

Conventional or CT angiography may demonstrate stenoses or aneurysms of visceral arteries without evidence of arteriosclerosis, FMD, or other noninflammatory causes (**162, 163**).

Electromyography (EMG) may be helpful in demonstrating neurological dysfunction, generally an axonal neuropathy, and is useful in guiding a biopsy.

Biopsy of an affected organ is the gold-standard for making a diagnosis. Biopsies should be guided by organ involvement, as 'blind' biopsies are associated with a high false-negative rate. Sural nerve and skin are common sites of biopsy. A skin biopsy must also contain subcutaneous fat (necessary to evaluate medium-sized blood vessels). The kidneys may be biopsied, but are associated with a high risk of hemorrhage due to the high frequency of aneurysms of the renal vasculature.

HISTOLOGY

The vessel walls in PAN demonstrate a patchy, transmural pleiomorphic cellular infiltrate with fibrinoid necrosis of the vessel wall. Involvement of the elastic lamina may lead to aneurysm development. Inflammation and intimal proliferation may lead to luminal narrowing.

PROGNOSIS

Untreated, PAN is nearly universally fatal, with a 5-year survival of only 13%. However, with treatment, the 5-year survival increases to 80%. A major cause of death is mesenteric infarction, cerebral infarction, and renal failure. The prognosis worsens as the number of organ systems involved increases. A prognostic index has been proposed to help predict mortality in PAN (*Table 56*). If none of these factors is present, the 5-year mortality is 12%, which increases to 46% if two or more criteria are present.

MANAGEMENT

GCs are the mainstay of treatment and alone may induce remission in up to 50% of patients. For severe disease, a combination of GCs (1 mg/kg of prednisone equivalent) with CTX is used. Generally, after induction of remission following 3–6 months of intensive therapy, a maintenance drug such as AZA is substituted for the CTX. Alternatives to CTX may be considered in patients in whom CTX is contraindicated or in less severe disease, and include chlorambucil, AZA, MTX, dapsone, cyclosporine, and plasma exchange. These agents have not been rigorously tested, and their efficacy is largely based on case reports and anecdotal data. For isolated cutaneous PAN, MTX may be effective. PAN associated with HBV is treated with a regimen consisting of lamivudine, prednisone, and plasma exchange.

Table 55 American College of Rheumatology classification criteria of polyarteritis nodosa, 1990*

Criterion

1. Weight loss of more than 4 kg
2. Livedo reticularis
3. Testicular pain or tenderness
4. Myalgias, weakness, or polyneuropathy
5. Mononeuropathy or multiple mononeuropathies
6. Diastolic blood pressure >90 mmHg
7. Elevated BUN or creatinine
8. Hepatitis B infection
9. Arteriographic abnormality
10. Biopsy of small- or medium- sized artery containing PMNs

* Polyarteritis nodosa diagnosis requires presence of three or more criteria for classification purposes. PMN: polymorphonuclear cell.

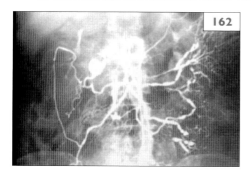

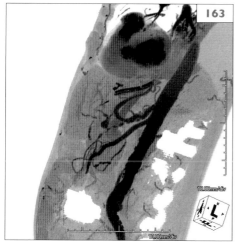

162, 163 Abdominal mesenteric angiograms in separate patients with PAN showing multiple vessels with segmental narrowing and poststenotic dilatation (arrow). (Courtesy of Dr GF Moore.)

Table 56 Prognostic index in polyarteritis nodosa*; 5 factor score

Proteinuria >1 g/day
Serum creatinine >1.6 mg/dl (>141 μmol/l)
Cardiomyopathy
Gastrointestinal involvement
Central nervous system involvement

*5-year mortality: 12% if no factors present *vs.* 5-year mortality: 46% if ≥2 factors present

Immune complex-mediated small-vessel vasculitis

DEFINITION

The inflammatory changes occurring in many forms of small-vessel vasculitis result from the deposition of immune complexes in the vessel wall. The immune complex (IC)-mediated small-vessel vasculitides include hypersensitivity vasculitis, Henoch–Schönlein purpura (HSP), mixed cryoglobulinemia (MC, most often associated with HCV infection), urticarial vasculitis, erythema elevatum diutinum, and vasculitides secondary to CTDs, including RA and SLE. Specific characteristics of hypersensitivity vasculitis, HSP, and MC will be discussed separately as they are three of the most commonly encountered forms of IC-mediated small-vessel vasculitis; features common to all IC vasculitides will first be discussed.

EPIDEMIOLOGY AND ETIOLOGY

ICs (combination of antigen with antibody) are normally cleared by the reticuloendothelial system. However, in circumstances of slight antigen excess, the ICs precipitate from the serum and may deposit into the vascular beds. Vasculitis results when these ICs deposit within the vessel walls leading to complement fixation, recruitment of neutrophils, release of degradative enzymes, generation of free radicals, and an ensuing local inflammatory reaction. Thrombus formation and hemorrhagic infarction may also occur. Although relatively uncommon as a group, hypersensitivity vasculitis is the most commonly encountered form of small-vessel vasculitis.

CLINICAL HISTORY AND PHYSICAL EXAMINATION

The small blood vessels are located primarily within the superficial papillary dermis. Given the superficial location of the vessels, it is not surprising that IC-mediated vasculitis of these vessels results in cutaneous manifestations. Palpable purpura is a hallmark of small-vessel vasculitides, and is most common in those mediated by IC deposition (**164**). These lesions result from the extravasation of red blood cells through inflamed and porous vessel walls into surrounding tissue. Purpuric lesions are generally found on dependent regions (especially lower legs) and are typically symmetrically distributed. They do not blanch with pressure and may result in hyperpigmentation of the affected skin following resolution.

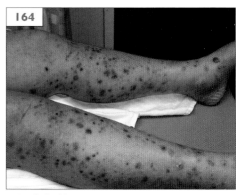

164 Palpable purpura in a patient with Henoch-Schönlein purpura. Note the symmetric distribution and involvement of the lower extremities. (Courtesy of Dr GF Moore.)

INVESTIGATIONS

Biopsy of the affected skin is paramount in the evaluation of cutaneous vasculitides. Biopsies should be performed on nonulcerated lesions (or from the ulcer's edge). Both examination under light microscopy and direct immunofluorescence (DIF) is crucial in order to characterize accurately the type of vasculitis, as ICs are not demonstrated with light microscopy alone. Because DIF requires fresh tissue (not formalin fixed), two separate biopsies are often required. Depending on the clinical picture, other potentially helpful tests may include serum chemistries, CBC, UA, HCV antibody, serum cryoglobulins, HIV serology, RF, anticitrullinated peptide antibody (anti-CCP), ANA, and serum complements. Inflammatory markers (including ESR and CRP) may be elevated in select cases and may track with treatment response.

HISTOLOGY

Cutaneous vasculitis classically demonstrates disruption of the blood vessel architecture with infiltrate of inflammatory cells within and near the vessel walls. This histopathologic finding is often termed leukocytoclastic vasculitis. On DIF, the staining pattern of fluorescein-labeled antibodies (anti-IgG, IgM, IgA, C3, and others) may allow for further characterization of the specific type of vasculitis.

Henoch–Schönlein purpura

DEFINITION
HSP is a vasculitis affecting small blood vessels and is associated with deposition of ICs containing IgA, characterized clinically by arthritic, cutaneous, and GI manifestations.

EPIDEMIOLOGY AND ETIOLOGY
HSP is primarily a childhood disease with a median age of 4 years. The incidence of HSP ranges from 10 to 20 per 100 000 in children. Approximately one-half of cases are preceded by an upper respiratory illness, and there is seasonal variation in disease incidence, with higher incidence in spring months in North America and Europe. The etiology of HSP is incompletely understood. Infectious and medication-related triggers have been proposed, but none have been proven.

CLINICAL HISTORY AND PHYSICAL EXAMINATION
While HSP is classically characterized by the triad of: 1) purpura; 2) colicky abdominal pain; and 3) arthritis; renal, genitourinary, and pulmonary manifestations are also seen:
- Nonthrombocytopenic, palpable purpura is generally seen on dependent areas, such as the buttocks and lower extremities.
- Early in the disease course, painful edema of the hands, ears, feet, and scalp may occur.
- The arthritis, which is less prevalent in adult-onset HSP, has a predilection for lower extremity large joints (typically knees and ankles) and is generally self-limited and nonerosive.
- GI involvement occurs in up to 85% of patients, and may manifest as colicky abdominal pain, nausea, vomiting, GI bleeding, bowel wall edema, and rarely intussusception.
- Renal manifestations occur in 10–50% of children with HSP, but up to 45–85% of adults with HSP. Renal involvement typically occurs within 3 months of the onset of purpura, and generally has a favorable outcome. HSP accounts for only 5% of children with chronic kidney disease (CKD) and 1% of end-stage renal disease (ESRD) in

children. However, renal outcomes are not as favorable in adult-onset HSP, with up to 30% having CKD. HSP accounts for fewer than 2% of adult glomerulonephritides.
- Other manifestations, such as testicular pain and acute scrotal swelling, thought to result from vasculitis of the testicular vessels, have also been reported. While pulmonary involvement in HSP is less commonly reported, interstitial pneumonias and diffuse alveolar hemorrhage can occur rarely. Interestingly, reversible decreases in diffusion capacities are seen in HSP, and thought to be a reflection of altered alveolar–capillary membranes due to circulating ICs. It has been postulated that this may be a useful measure of disease activity in select patients.

DIFFERENTIAL DIAGNOSIS
The differential diagnosis of HSP is largely guided by organ involvement, but in general, includes hypersensitivity vasculitis, acute hemorrhagic edema of childhood, cryoglobulinemia, juvenile idiopathic arthritis (JIA), SLE, or other systemic vasculitides.

INVESTIGATIONS
HSP is primarily a clinical diagnosis, with no diagnostic studies or laboratory tests *per se* required for diagnosis. Appropriate laboratory investigations should be done to evaluate for renal involvement (UA, creatinine, urine protein/creatinine ratio), and to exclude other entities within the differential. Elevated serum IgA is consistent with, but not diagnostic of HSP. A skin or kidney biopsy may be necessary if the diagnosis is in question, and many advocate for a kidney biopsy if there is evidence of significant renal involvement (see Histology overleaf). Kidney biopsy with renal involvement is consistent with IgA nephropathy. Because IgA does not activate complement, serum C3 and C4 levels are typically normal. Select use of imaging studies may be required for the evaluation of pulmonary and/or abdominal symptoms.

HISTOLOGY
Hematoxylin and eosin staining of skin biopsies in HSP demonstrate a leukocytoclastic vasculitis and

IgA and C3 along small vessels is demonstrated on immunofluorescent staining (**165, 166**). In HSP, diffuse deposition of IgA, C3, properidin, fibrin, and IgM are seen on immunofluorescent staining of kidney biopsies and mesangial, subendothelial, and subepithelial deposits are demonstrated on electron microscopy.

PROGNOSIS
Most cases (especially pediatric HSP) resolve without complication. However, some patients (mostly adults) will have a chronic disease course. Less than 5% of children with HSP will have CKD, and <1% will progress to ESRD. However, up to 30% of adults with HSP will have CKD. Poor prognostic features include nephrotic range proteinuria, as 15% of these will progress to ESRD.

MANAGEMENT
Treatment of HSP is generally supportive. Analgesics and nonsteroidal anti-inflammatory drugs (NSAIDs) generally benefit the arthralgias, though caution is warranted with NSAIDs in those with renal dysfunction. Steroids may be beneficial for the painful edema seen in early disease. Data are conflicting as to whether corticosteroid treatment prevents development of nephritis and this treatment is not currently recommended. If nephritis is present, high-dose corticosteroids are recommended, and pulse CTX has also demonstrated efficacy. Other treatments such as plasma exchange, AZA, cyclosporine, IVIG, and others have been used, but are not recommended as first-line therapy. Aggressive treatment of nephritis may alter disease progression.

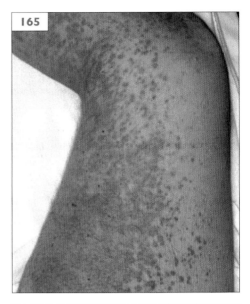

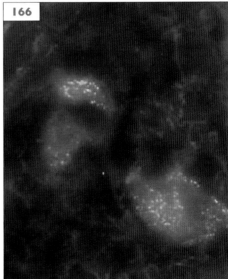

165, 166 Skin involvement in a patient with Henoch-Schönlein purpura (**165**) and corresponding biopsy with direct immunofluorescence demonstrating IgA deposition (**166**). (With permission from the American College of Rheumatology.)

Hypersensitivity vasculitis

DEFINITION
Hypersensitivity vasculitis is an inflammatory disorder of small blood vessels mediated by IC deposition following an exposure (usually a drug or infection) and spares the internal organs.

EPIDEMIOLOGY AND ETIOLOGY
Hypersensitivity vasculitis is the most common form of IC-mediated small vessel vasculitis.

Exposures which can trigger the development of hypersensitivity vasculitis are most commonly drugs (penicillins, cephalosporins, sulfonamides, phenytoin, and allopurinol) or infections (HBV, HCV, chronic bacteremia). In approximately one-half of all cases, no inciting exposure is identified.

CLINICAL HISTORY AND PHYSICAL EXAMINATION
Hypersensitivity vasculitis presents similar to other IC-mediated small-vessel vasculitides, with palpable purpura and other cutaneous manifestations (**167**). The key feature in distinguishing it from other vasculitides is its lack of visceral involvement and the temporal relationship with an inciting exposure. However, because nearly one-half of cases do not have an identifiable inciting exposure, hypersensitivity vasculitis is often a diagnosis of exclusion.

INVESTIGATIONS
As previously mentioned, skin biopsy is paramount in the evaluation of any unexplained cutaneous vasculitis. No laboratory tests are diagnostic of hypersensitivity vasculitis and are undertaken primarily to exclude other systemic disorders which may present similarly.

PROGNOSIS
In most cases of hypersensitivity vasculitis, the prognosis is excellent without significant detrimental effects on morbidity or mortality.

MANAGEMENT
The management of hypersensitivity vasculitis consists primarily of removing the offending agent or treating the underlying disease. In some instances, patients may experience repeated flares, and may benefit from low-dose GCs, dapsone, or colchicine as suppressive therapy.

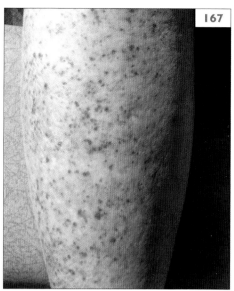

167 Lower extremity purpura in a patient with hypersensitivity vasculitis. (Courtesy of Dr GF Moore.)

Mixed cryoglobulinemia

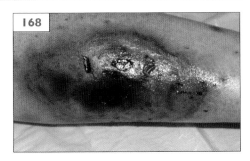

DEFINITION
Cryoglobulins are circulating immunoglobulins which precipitate at temperatures less than 37°C. MC consists of polyclonal IgG and either monoclonal (type II) or polyclonal IgM (type III). A small-vessel vasculitis may result when the resulting ICs, antigen, and complement are deposited within the vessel wall.

EPIDEMIOLOGY AND ETIOLOGY
Infections, especially HCV, are the most common inciting event leading to development of MC. Other infections, such as HIV, and autoimmune disorders, namely Sjögren's syndrome (SS), have also been identified as triggers. Approximately 30–50% of patients with HCV will have detectable serum cryoglobulins, though a very small minority (up to 5%) will develop symptoms. When an underlying disorder is not identified, the disorder is described as 'essential' cryoglobulinemia. The overall incidence of MC is not known.

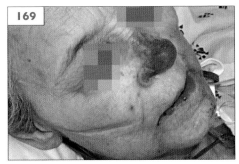

CLINICAL HISTORY AND PHYSICAL EXAMINATION
Dermatologic, musculoskeletal and neurologic manifestations of cryoglobulinemic vasculitis are most common, though multiple systems may also be involved (**168–170**).
- Dermatologic: Petechial or palpable purpuric lesions (typically of dependent areas or distal digits, nose, ears) are most common and may progress to ulcerations (**168, 169**).
- Musculoskeletal: Arthralgias are common in MC, though true arthritis is rare. When present, the arthritis of MC generally involves medium and large joints, and is nonerosive.
- Neurologic: Peripheral neuropathy is a frequent manifestation of MC, and most commonly presents as a mild sensory neuritis. Less frequently, a more severe neuropathy with or without motor involvement may occur (**170**).
- Renal: Membrano-proliferative glomerulonephritis (MPGN) may occur in MC, and often has significant implications on prognosis and survival.

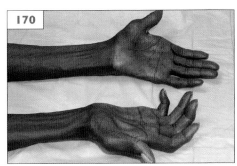

168–170 Findings with mixed cryoglobulinemia related to chronic hepatitis C virus infection. **168**: Ulcerative lesions in lower extremity; **169**: marked cyanosis of nose; **170**: severe muscle wasting in patient with diffuse neuropathy secondary to mixed cryoglobulinemia.

- Pulmonary: Interstitial lung disease (ILD) and alveolitis have been reported in MC, though the exact relationship of these manifestations is unclearly defined.
- Endocrine: Autoimmune thyroiditis, thyroid cancer, and hypothyroidism are over-represented in MC, relative to the general population.
- GI: Rarely MC may manifest as intestinal vasculitis and mimic a surgical abdomen.
- Hematologic: B cell malignancies may occur as a late complication of MC.

INVESTIGATIONS

The diagnosis of MC requires the presence of circulating cryoglobulins, though the severity of disease does not correlate with the level of circulating cryoglobulins. Serum RF is almost universally present in MC, and serum complements (especially C4) are often low. Other serologic evaluations depend on the presenting features, but often include those focused on working up an undifferentiated vasculitis: ANCA, ANA, UA, chest X-ray, EMG, and other appropriate tests. A skin biopsy usually shows leukocytoclastic vasculitis. Once cryoglobulinemia is diagnosed, attempts to identify an underlying cause should be performed, namely evaluating for HCV (or other chronic infections) and auto-immune disorders (especially primary SS).

PROGNOSIS

The prognosis of patients with MC is variable, depending on extent and severity of organ involvement as well as responsiveness to therapy. Renal involvement has been associated with a worse prognosis. The mean 10-year survival (after diagnosis) is 50–60%.

MANAGEMENT

The decision to treat MC should be based on symptoms of vasculitis rather than simply on the presence of circulating cryoglobulins, as many of these patients are asymptomatic. The initial treatment of MC should target the underlying disorder. In HCV-associated MC, treatment with antiviral therapy (e.g. IFN and ribavirin) is indicated. In patients with 'essential' MC, rituximab or CTX is considered the primary therapy. Low-dose corticosteroids may be beneficial in the treatment of the dermatologic manifestations, arthralgias, weakness, and mild sensory neuropathy. Other immunosuppressive therapies (CTX, rituximab) and plasma exchange may be necessary for severe or refractory manifestations. Though formal guidelines have not been developed, patients with MC should be monitored periodically for development of B cell malignancies.

Kawasaki's disease

DEFINITION
Kawasaki's disease (KD) is a vasculitis, primarily affecting children under 5 years of age, and is characterized by fevers, cutaneous and oropharyngeal manifestations, and cardiovascular involvement. KD has also been referred to as 'mucocutaneous lymph node syndrome'.

EPIDEMIOLOGY AND ETIOLOGY
KD is relatively rare with an incidence of 100–150 cases per 100 000 children under 5 years of age. The peak age of onset is 1 year, and 80–85% of cases occur prior to age 5 years. A slight male to female predominance exists (1.4:1). Although KD is seen worldwide, it is most prevalent in developed countries. The highest prevalence is seen in those of Japanese ancestry with the lowest frequency in Caucasians. Seasonal variation has been described in both Japan and the US and occasionally occurs in pandemics. The etiology of KD is not well understood although there is substantial speculation regarding the causal role of a yet identified infectious agent. The increased predisposition for KD observed in Asian populations suggests that genetic risk factors may also play a role.

PATHOGENESIS
The immune system in KD becomes activated leading to release of proinflammatory cytokines (TNF-α, IFN-γ, IL-1, IL-4, IL-6, and IL-10), activation of complement and IC deposition. The inflammatory cascade ultimately results in weakening of the vessel endothelium leading to formation of aneurysms. Aneurysmal formation has been shown to correlate with serum levels of TNF-α. The predilection by KD for involvement of the coronary vessels is not well understood, but may be related to activation of endothelial cells and the production of antiendothelial cell antibodies.

CLINICAL HISTORY AND PHYSICAL EXAMINATION
Like most vasculitides, KD has multisystemic manifestations. KD is characterized by:
- High fevers: Abrupt onset; may last 5 days or more.
- Bilateral nonpurulent conjunctival congestion occurs within 2–4 days of fever onset.
- Painful cervical lymphadenopathy shortly prior to or after the onset of fevers.
- Oropharyngeal manifestations: erythema, drying, and fissuring of lips; erythema of the tongue ('strawberry tongue').
- Exanthem: trunk and extremities 1–5 days after fever onset.
- Palmar and plantar erythema.
- Desquamative rash, starting in the periungual regions; 10–15 days following the fever.
- Irritability and behavioral changes.
- Cardiac manifestations: Coronary aneurysms, carditis, myocardial infarction.
- Arthritis: 20–30%.
- GI manifestations: Nausea, vomiting, mild transaminase elevation, jaundice.
- 'Cytokine storm' Severe KD; due to increased production of proinflammatory cytokines; may result in a macrophage activation syndrome.

Diagnostic criteria have been proposed to aid in the identification of KD, though patients who do not satisfy these criteria may be considered to have 'incomplete KD' (*Table 57*).

DIFFERENTIAL DIAGNOSIS
The differential diagnosis for KD is broad. A variety of infections may mimic KD and need to be excluded. Frequently, viral exanthems of childhood closely mimic KD. Other entities which closely resemble KD include streptococcal scarlet fever, Stevens–Johnson syndrome, systemic juvenile-onset inflammatory arthritis, and toxic shock syndrome. A diagnosis of KD needs to be considered in all pediatric patients presenting with spiking fevers for at least 4 days which are not otherwise explained.

INVESTIGATIONS
KD is a clinical diagnosis. As such, most of the laboratory investigations which are performed are done to exclude other etiologies, primarily infectious diseases. Commonly, patients with KD will have a mild leukocytosis with left shift, elevated acute phase reactants, negative antistreptolysin O titers, negative pharyngeal cultures, mild elevations of hepatic transaminases, and pleiocytosis of the cerebrospinal fluid. Transthoracic echocardiography should be done at diagnosis and weekly for 1 month thereafter to assess for cardiac involvement and aneurysm formation.

HISTOLOGY

Histological evaluation of involved blood vessels in KD reveals a nonspecific inflammatory arteritis similar to that of PAN seen in adults.

PROGNOSIS

Generally KD is a self-limited disorder, though it can be associated with long-term cardiovascular complications. In the absence of cardiac complications, long-term morbidity and mortality related to KD are negligible. With prompt diagnosis and treatment, the long-term manifestations which affect a small percentage of patients, can be prevented. Overall, the mortality for KD is low, 0.1–0.3% of all cases, and usually results from thrombosis of coronary vessels. Of deaths from KD, males outnumber females three to one.

MANAGEMENT

Management of KD consists primarily of supportive care, IVIG, and ASA. Antibiotics do not have a role in the management of KD, and corticosteroids are not recommended due to concerns that they may hasten aneurysmal formation. IVIG (2g/kg) and ASA (80–100 mg/kg/day) are effective in reducing the development of aneurysms and have become the standard of care for patients with KD. Often, a single dose of IVIG is sufficient. However, if fevers recur, retreatment may be done. In refractory cases of KD, infliximab has been shown to be effective. Pentoxifylline has also shown promise in the management of KD, in improving clinical outcomes and reducing the development of aneurysms. Anticoagulation may be warranted in select cases to prevent thrombi in large coronary aneurysms.

Table 57 Principal critieria for the diagnosis of Kawasaki's disease (5 of 6 critieria required)

- Fever lasting ≥4 days
- Bilateral nonpurulent conjunctival injection
- Changes of the lips and oral cavity (fissuring, cracking,strawberry tongue, reddening of oral mucosa
- Polymorphous rash (typically truncal)
- Acute nonpurulent lymphadenopathy (cervical node ≥1.5 cm)
- Dermatologic changes of distal extremities (reddening of palms/soles, desquamative changes of finger tips, indurative edema of hands/feet

Thromboangiitis obliterans (Buerger's disease)

DEFINITION
Thromboangiitis obliterans (TAO) is a nonatherosclerotic, inflammatory, vaso-occlusive disorder which primarily affects the distal extremities and occurs almost exclusively in smokers.

EPIDEMIOLOGY AND ETIOLOGY
TAO is rare and has a male predilection. It occurs worldwide, but is more prevalent in the Middle East, Asia, and Mediterranean areas. The development of TAO is strongly associated with nicotine use, especially cigarette smoking. No substantiated cases of TAO have been reported in patients who did not use nicotine. Recently, the incidence in North America has been declining, which is thought to be related to decreasing smoking rates. The onset of TAO is variable but most frequently affects those less than 40–45 years of age. No genetic risk factors for the development of TAO have been discovered.

The etiology of TAO is not well understood. Although the association of TAO with tobacco use is well described, the mechanism by which this triggers the disease process has not been elucidated. Endothelial dysfunction is a key feature of TAO as impaired endothelial-dependent vasodilation has been demonstrated, even in unaffected limbs in patients with TAO. It has been proposed that TAO is an autoimmune phenomenon with its manifestations resulting from an immunological response to nicotine, although this remains unproven.

PATHOGENESIS
The pathogenesis of TAO is incompletely understood. It has been proposed that the inciting event in the development of TAO may be mechanical injury which in concert with a dysregulated immune system and environmental factors, such as smoking, accelerates the development of intimal lesions. Fibrinolytic activity is thought to be decreased within the thickened intima and may contribute to the development of occlusive thrombosis.

CLINICAL HISTORY AND PHYSICAL EXAMINATION
The initial manifestations of TAO may be subtle, including mild paresthesias and pain in hands and feet with exposure to the cold. This may rapidly evolve to severe claudication (pain elicited with activity), digital ischemia, splinter hemorrhages, cyanosis, digital ulceration, and intense pain (**171**). The vascular territories involved in TAO are generally those of small arteries and veins in distal extremities, though reports of involvement of the coronary, mesenteric, and pulmonary vasculature exist. Superficial thrombophlebitis is seen in approximately one-third of patients. An abnormal Allen's test in a young patient with lower extremity ulcers is suggestive of TAO. Although a relatively sensitive test, the Allen's test may be abnormal in other conditions such as scleroderma (SSc).

To perform an Allen's Test:
- The patient is asked to make a fist ('emptying' blood flow from fingers).
- The examiner holds the thumbs across thenar and hypothenar eminence to occlude radial and ulnar arteries.
- The patient then opens the hand; pressure on the ulnar artery is released while radial artery occlusion is maintained.
- The test is subsequently repeated, releasing pressure on the radial artery and maintaining an occluded ulnar artery.

In a normal test, blood flow returns promptly to the digits after removal of pressure from one artery; with an abnormal test result, there is persistent palor in the digits following removal of pressure.

DIFFERENTIAL DIAGNOSIS
The differential diagnosis of TAO is broad, but includes other vasculitides and vasculopathies. Consideration should be given to the possibility of atherosclerotic disease, embolic phenomena, arteritis, SSc, hyperviscosity syndromes, ergot toxicity, toxindromes, and hypercoagulable conditions when evaluating patients for TAO.

Diagnostic criteria for TAO include:
- Lower extremity ischemia in a young smoker (e.g. <45 years of age) with at least two of the following:
  - Superficial thrombophlebitis.

- Arterial upper limb involvement.
- Raynaud's phenomenon.

These criteria assume that other mimics (diabetes mellitus, atherosclerotic vascular disease, autoimmune disease including scleroderma, hypercoagulable states, embolic disease) are excluded.

INVESTIGATIONS

No specific laboratory tests are diagnostic of TAO, and most of the investigations are aimed at excluding other entities:

- Inflammatory markers are typically normal.
- RF, ANA, Scl-70 antibodies, anticentromere antibodies, and antiphospholipid antibodies (aPLs) are generally absent.
- Screening for cocaine, amphetamines, and cannabis should be performed as appropriate as these drugs can cause a clinical and radiographic picture indistinguishable from TAO.
- Cardiac source of emboli should be excluded with echocardiography.
- Angiography reveals multiple areas of bilateral narrowing or occlusion in the digital, plantar, palmar, radial, ulnar, peroneal, and tibial arteries (**172**); 'corkscrew' collaterals are often seen, but are not pathognomonic; proximal vasculature should appear otherwise normal without atherosclerosis.

HISTOLOGY

Biopsy, while not routinely performed, demonstrates a segmental inflammatory response with highly cellular thrombosis and microabscesses in acutely affected blood vessels. The intimal elastic lamina is preserved and the degree of inflammatory cell infiltrate within the vessel wall is less than with other vasculitides. In chronic TAO, there may be little inflammatory infiltrate with more organized thrombus and secondary fibrosis.

PROGNOSIS

With successful smoking cessation and avoidance of other forms of tobacco, the prognosis in TAO is generally favorable. A vast majority of patients who successfully quit smoking avoid amputation. If nicotine use continues, approximately 50% of patients will require amputation.

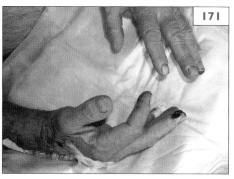

171 Ischemic ulcerations of distal digits in a patient with thromboangiitis obliterans. (Courtesy of Dr GF Moore.)

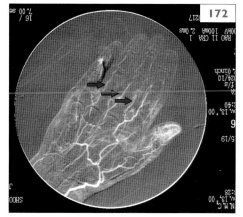

172 Conventional angiography of the hand demonstrating narrowing and tapering of multiple digital arteries and extensive collateralization, most prominent in distal thumb. (Courtesy of Dr GF Moore.)

MANAGEMENT

The most important intervention in TAO is complete nicotine cessation and avoidance of all other tobacco products. Use of nicotine replacement therapy may actually protract the disease course and should therefore be avoided if possible. Avoidance of 'second-hand' exposure to smoke is also paramount. Measurement of serum or urine cotinine (a by-product of nicotine) may be useful in monitoring adherence to cessation programs. Wound care plays a crucial role in the management of ischemic lesions due to TAO, to prevent secondary infections.

Dihydropyridine calcium channel blockers (e.g. nifedipine, amlodipine) may be used to help combat vasospasm, and cilastazol may help with improving perfusion of ischemic areas, thus promoting healing of ulcerations. Other therapies which may have a role include ASA, prostaglandin analogues such as iloprost, pentoxifylline, and intra-arterial streptokinase.

Surgical revascularization may be beneficial in select patients and amputation is recommended as a last resort. Sympathectomy has not been shown to play a pivotal role in the management of TAO.

Primary angiitis of the central nervous system

DEFINITION

Primary angiitis of the central nervous system (PACNS) is a rare and heterogeneous disorder characterized by inflammation of the blood vessels (vasculitis) and is isolated to the vasculature of the CNS.

EPIDEMIOLOGY AND ETIOLOGY

PACNS may affect all ages with a mean age at diagnosis of 42 years, and is thought to have a slight male predominance (2:1). Owing to the rarity of this entity, the incidence and prevalence are not well defined, though an incidence of ~8 cases per 1 000 000 person-years in Olmsted County, in the US, has been reported. Likewise, the etiopathogenesis of PACNS is not well understood. Infectious agents have been proposed to be etiologic in the development of PACNS, but no conclusive link has been found.

PATHOGENESIS

Given its rare nature, the pathogenesis of PACNS remains poorly defined.

CLINICAL HISTORY AND PHYSICAL EXAMINATION

PACNS generally presents subacutely, with both focal and diffuse neurologic dysfunction occurring over 3–6 months. The most common presenting features include headache, confusion, and mental status changes. Less common symptoms include TIAs, cerebrovascular accidents, paresis, visual changes, coma, encephalopathy, dementia, and seizures. Symptoms common to systemic vasculitides (fevers, weight loss, peripheral neuropathies, rashes) are uncommon.

DIFFERENTIAL DIAGNOSIS

Infections (VZV, syphilis, tuberculosis, brucellosis, and rickettsial disease), reversible cerebral vasoconstriction syndrome, and sarcoidosis are important conditions to exclude within the differential diagnosis of PACNS, but many other entities may mimic PACNS closely (*Table 58*). The diagnostic criteria for PACNS (see below) highlight the need to evaluate for, and exclude conditions which may mimic this disorder.

Diagnostic criteria proposed by Calabrese and Mallek in 1988 defined PACNS as:

The presence of an acquired and otherwise unexplained neurologic deficit after a thorough investigation with satisfaction of the following two criteria:

1 The presence of either classic angiographic or histological features of angiitis within the CNS,
   AND
2 No evidence of systemic vasculitis or any condition that could elicit the angiographic or pathologic changes.

INVESTIGATIONS

No laboratory abnormality is specific for PACNS. The most essential laboratory investigation involves a thorough evaluation for infectious mimics. Cerebrospinal fluid analysis should be obtained in each patient when PACNS is considered, and generally shows mild elevation in protein and white blood cell count, findings similar to aseptic meningitis. Inflammatory markers such as ESR and CRP are usually normal or only slightly elevated. ANAs, ANCAs, aPLs, and RF are generally negative, and if present, should prompt consideration of an alternate diagnosis.

While there are no radiographic changes specific for PACNS, several imaging modalities are useful in the evaluation for PACNS and in ruling out mimicking conditions (*Table 58*), including MRI or CT (with or without angiography) and conventional angiography. Several findings are consistent with the diagnosis including: cerebral perfusion defects, ischemic brain lesions, intracerebral or subarachnoid hemorrhages, vascular stenosis without evidence of atherosclerosis, and vessel wall thickening with contrast enhancement. MRI may be normal, but commonly shows multiple, bilateral cerebral lesions involving the deep white matter. Very rarely, PACNS may present as a solitary mass lesion. Cerebral angiography is of low specificity for PACNS as several entities may have identical angiographic features. Typical angiographic changes in PACNS involve smooth-walled segmental stenosis and dilatation with occlusion of multiple cerebral vessels in the absence of proximal atherosclerotic changes (**173**).

Biopsy remains the gold standard for diagnosis of PACNS. Location of biopsy should be guided by abnormalities seen on imaging. The leptomeninges should be biopsied as well as cortex as

Table 58 Conditions that may mimic primary angiitis of the central nervous system

Mimics of PACNS

- Infectious: HIV, TB, VZV, syphillis, brucellosis
- Coagulopathies: APS
- Neoplastic: Lymphomas (HD, NHL, intravascular B cell)
- Migraines
- Vasoconstriction syndromes: RCVS, sympathomimetics
- Severe HTN
- Atherosclerotic disease
- Other: Amyloid angiopathy, sarcoid, Moya-Moya

APS: antiphospholipid antibody syndrome; HD: Hodgkin's disease; HIV: human immunodeficiency virus; HTN: hypertension; NHL: non-Hodgkin's lymphoma; RCVS: reversible cerebral vasoconstriction syndrome; TB: tuberculosis; VZV: varicella zoster virus.

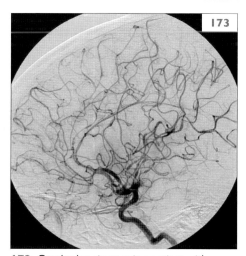

173 Cerebral angiogram in a patient with primary angiitis of the central nervous system. The angiogram demonstrates sequential narrowing and dilatation of cerebral arteries in a wide distribution. These angiographic findings are consistent with, but not diagnostic of, CNS vasculitis. Cerebral vasospasm may have a similar angiographic appearance. (With permission, American College of Rheumatology.)

it increases the diagnostic yield. Stereotactic approaches also increase the yield of the biopsy. Cerebral biopsy is diagnostic in 50–75% of cases, with false negatives owing to the segmental involvement of the vasculature.

HISTOLOGY

Three distinct histological patterns of PACNS (primarily involving small arteries and arterioles) have been described, although these patterns do not appear to impact overall prognosis:

- Granulomatous.
- Lymphocytic.
- Necrotizing.

PROGNOSIS

If untreated, PACNS may be a progressive and fatal disorder. There is a subset of patients who exhibit a more benign course. However, predicting which patients will follow a more favorable course is difficult. Features associated with a poor prognosis include: focal neurologic deficits, cognitive impairment, cerebrovascular accident, and large vessel involvement.

MANAGEMENT

There are no clinical trials of therapy for PACNS, and empiric treatment is based on experience with the treatment of other vasculitides. The current standard therapy consists of induction with CTX and high-dose GCs (initially 1–1.5 mg/kg/day of prednisone or its equivalent) for 3–6 months (over which time the steroids are slowly weaned to a low dose), followed by maintenance therapy with AZA or MTX. With early diagnosis and treatment, remission can be obtained in the majority of patients.

Other Rheumatic Conditions

- Osteoporosis
- Fibromyalgia and other soft tissue syndromes
- Sarcoidosis
- Amyloidosis
- Miscellaneous rheumatic conditions

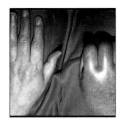
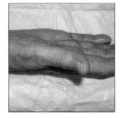
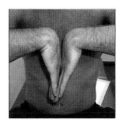
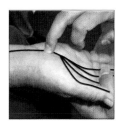

Osteoporosis

DEFINITION

Osteoporosis is a state of 'low bone mass', routinely measured using noninvasive densitometric techniques, accompanied by the disproportionate occurrence of characteristic fragility fractures.

EPIDEMIOLOGY AND ETIOLOGY

Osteoporosis leading to fracture represents a growing public health issue; a problem that is projected to increase with a rapidly aging population. It is estimated that there are more than 1.3 million osteoporosis-related fractures annually in the US. The lifetime risk of hip, vertebral, or wrist fracture (fracture sites most closely linked to osteoporosis) in a 50-year-old Caucasian woman is estimated to be approximately 40%, three times the corresponding risk in men. The proportion of postmenopausal women with osteoporosis varies based on age group, from ~15% in women 50–59 years of age to as high as 70% in women ≥80 years of age. In addition to female gender and older age, several other risk factors for osteoporosis and fracture have been identified (*Table 59*).

PATHOGENESIS

Bone structure, bone mineral density (BMD), and bone function are dependent on continual remodeling – new bone formation balanced with resorption. The cellular balance of bone-forming cells (osteoblasts) and bone-resorbing cells (osteoclasts) is referred to as 'coupling'. Osteoporosis is the result of excessive bone resorption at the expense of new bone formation.

CLINICAL HISTORY

A history of fragility fracture, particularly those involving the hip, spine, and wrist, should heighten suspicion and lead to an evaluation for underlying osteoporosis. A history of 'height loss' (more than 4 cm over 10 years) and/or subjective changes in posture could serve as clinical markers for osteoporosis. Individuals with a history of prior fracture in addition to women over 50 years and men over 60 years of age should be routinely screened for the presence of osteoporosis risk factors (*Table 59*).

PHYSICAL EXAMINATION

While the history and physical examination alone lack sensitivity in detecting osteoporosis, these remain important components of the overall patient evaluation. A major goal of the physical examination is to detect evidence of chronic disease that may contribute to accelerated bone loss (*Table 60*). A physical finding of kyphoscoliosis may be indicative of osteoporosis complicated by vertebral compression fracture (**174**).

DIFFERENTIAL DIAGNOSIS

Secondary causes of osteoporosis should be considered in the evaluation of patients with suspected osteoporosis or in the context of fragility

---

Table 59 Risk factors for osteoporosis and fracture

Sociodemographics and family history	Biologic measures	Health and behaviors
Race/ethnicity*	Low bone mass	Frequent falls
Older age	Low vitamin D levels	Glucocorticoid use
Female gender	Low body mass index	Decreased physical activity
Family history of osteoporosis	Hypogonadism or premature menopause	Cigarette smoking
		Excessive alcohol intake

*Fracture risk is consistently lower in African-Americans than non-Hispanic Caucasians; although not well defined, hip fracture rates in Asians appear to be intermediate to those of Caucasians and African-Americans; rates in Hispanic populations approach rates observed for African-Americans.

fracture (*Table 60*). In addition to the causes of secondary osteoporosis listed in *Table 60*, other conditions can lead to pathologic fracture (e.g. osteomyeltis, malignancy) and should be ruled out in the appropriate clinical setting.

INVESTIGATIONS

Dual-energy X-ray absorptiometry (DXA) is currently the cornerstone of BMD measurement. In postmenopausal women, the World Health Organization (WHO) has defined osteoporosis to mean a BMD value that is more than 2.5 standard deviations (SDs) below the peak mean BMD in younger women. 'Osteopenia' refers to BMD values that are more than 1.0 SD below the peak BMD but do not reach the threshold of osteoporosis. DXA reports include site-specific absolute BMD (g/cm^2) in addition to corresponding T- (SD difference between patient and peak BMD in a reference population, typically younger women) and Z-scores (SD difference between patient and age-

Table 60 Secondary causes of osteoporosis

Endocrine/metabolic	Medications
Acromegaly	Exogenous glucocorticoids
Anorexia nervosa	Exogenous thyroid hormone
Secondary amenorrhea	Antiepileptics
Type I diabetes mellitus	Phenobarbital
Hyperthyroidism (primary or secondary)	Phenytoin
Cushing syndrome	Phenothiazines
Hemochromatosis	Heparin (prolonged administration)
Hyperparathyroidism	Gonadotrophin releasing hormone agonists
Low vitamin D	Cyclosporine
Collagen/genetic	**Neoplastic**
Ehlers–Danlos syndrome	Multiple myeloma
Glycogen storage diseases	
Marfan's syndrome	**Autoimmune**
Homocystinuria	Rheumatoid arthritis
Hypophosphatasia	
Osteogenesis imperfecta	**Malabsorption**
	Gastric bypass
	Celiac disease
	Other conditions causing malabsorption

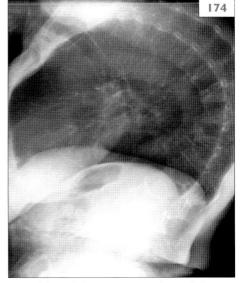

174 A lateral thoracic spine radiograph from an elderly woman with long-standing rheumatoid arthritis and a history of chronic prednisone use, demonstrating severe osteopenia, multiple thoracic compression fractures, and severe kyphosis. Corresponding lumbar spine bone mineral density, measured by dual energy X-ray absorptiometry, revealed a T-score of –4.4 standard deviations from peak young adult value. (Courtesy of Dr GF Moore.)

and sex-matched population) (**175**). Spine BMD may be falsely increased due to degenerative spine disease, particularly in older patients. Serial DXA plays an important role in reassessments of risk over time (generally repeated no sooner than every 1–2 years) and in monitoring treatment effect.

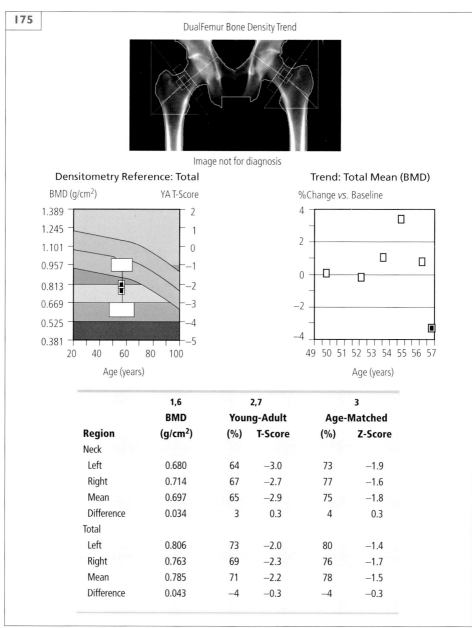

		1,6	**2,7**		**3**	
	BMD	**Young-Adult**		**Age-Matched**	
Region	**(g/cm²)**	**(%)**	**T-Score**	**(%)**	**Z-Score**
Neck					
Left	0.680	64	−3.0	73	−1.9
Right	0.714	67	−2.7	77	−1.6
Mean	0.697	65	−2.9	75	−1.8
Difference	0.034	3	0.3	4	0.3
Total					
Left	0.806	73	−2.0	80	−1.4
Right	0.763	69	−2.3	76	−1.7
Mean	0.785	71	−2.2	78	−1.5
Difference	0.043	−4	−0.3	−4	−0.3

175 Dual energy X-ray absorptiometry report showing osteoporotic range bone mineral density (BMD) of the femoral neck (mean T-score of −2.9) and osteopenic range BMD in the total hip (mean T-score of −2.2).

DXA measurement of alternative anatomic sites (heel or midradius) may play a role in select patients, but these measures are generally considered less informative than hip or spine measurements.

Recent emphasis has been placed on estimates of absolute fracture risk. The FRAX® tool, available online (www.shef.ac.uk/ FRAX/), was recently developed by the WHO to evaluate long-term (10-year) fracture risk of patients. FRAX® models are based on data from population-based cohorts and risks are computed based on BMD values and 11 other clinical variables (age, gender, weight, height, prior fracture, family history of fracture, current smoking, glucocorticoid [GC] use, rheumatoid arthritis [RA], secondary osteoporosis, and alcohol intake).

Laboratory evaluations are generally useful in ruling out secondary causes for osteoporosis (*Table 60*) and may include:
- Complete blood count (CBC).
- Serum chemistries including calcium, phosphorous, creatinine, glucose, albumin, and liver function tests.
- 25-OH vitamin D.
- Endocrine studies including thyroid stimulating hormone (TSH) and intact parathyroid hormone level (iPTH).
- Serum protein electrophoresis.

Other laboratories may be appropriate based on clues from the history and physical examination suggesting alternative secondary causes for bone loss. The role of bone turnover markers (e.g. bone-specific alkaline phosphatase, urine/serum N- or C-telopeptide) in the diagnosis and management of osteoporosis remains controversial. These tests may play an important role only in select circumstances, and may be reasonable indicators of treatment adherence relatively early in the course of osteoporosis treatment.

Radiography and advanced imaging techniques (magnetic resonance imaging [MRI], computed tomography [CT]) play an important role in detecting fragility fracture in patients with osteopenia and osteoporosis.

HISTOLOGY

Although the diagnosis of osteoporosis is typically made using noninvasive techniques, bone biopsy may be indicated in rare cases. Most often, this involves biopsy of the iliac crest and is used to exclude the possibility of alternative metabolic bone diseases. In addition to routine histological evaluation, histomorphometric parameters of the sampled bone may be assessed (cancellous bone volume, osteoid volume, osteoid surface, and resorption [eroded] surface). Dynamic evaluations using labeled tetracycline may provide additional information about the cellular components of sampled bone. Osteoporotic bone is characterized by a reduction in trabecular bone volume in addition to important differences in bone microstructure, most notably discontinuity in the trabecular lattice due to erosion by osteoclasts.

PROGNOSIS

Fragility fractures have a major detrimental impact on morbidity and mortality. It has been estimated that both hip and vertebral fractures are associated with an overall reduction in survival of 10–20%. Likewise, following hip fracture, approximately one-half of patients are unable to walk without assistance and approximately one-third become totally dependent. These data underscore the importance of primary and secondary fracture prevention.

MANAGEMENT

Strategies of prevention, particularly in those with prior fracture or in postmenopausal women or men over age 65 years, should be considered:
- Weight-bearing exercise.
- Smoking cessation.
- Optimize nutritional status (calcium and vitamin D supplementation).
- Addressing and correcting modifiable secondary causes of bone loss.
- Bisphosphonates should be considered for prevention of osteoporosis in patients taking chronic GCs (prednisone dose of 5–7.5 mg/ day or greater).

The National Osteoporosis Foundation (NOF) currently recommends treatment of osteoporosis for patients if any one of the following criteria are met:
- History of hip or vertebral fracture.
- A T-score of ≤−2.5 at the femoral neck, total hip, or spine.
- Low BMD (osteopenia or worse) and FRAX 10-year absolute hip fracture risk exceeding 3%.
- Low BMD and FRAX 10-year absolute risk of other major osteoporotic risk fracture exceeding 20%.

Bisphosphonates remain the cornerstone of osteoporosis treatment. Approved bisphosphonates include alendronate (daily or weekly PO), residronate (daily or weekly PO), ibandronate (monthly PO/IV), and zoledronic acid (yearly IV). Bisphosphonates have been shown to retard BMD loss over time and significantly reduce fracture risk. They are effective in the treatment of primary osteoporosis and in the treatment/prevention of GC-induced osteoporosis (GIOP). Contraindications to bisphosphonate use include hypersensitivity to the drug or one of its components, hypocalcemia, pregnancy, and severe renal dysfunction (creatinine clearance ≤30 mg/min). Caution should be used in the use of oral bisphosphonates in patients with mechanical problems of the esophagus (stricture, dysmotility) or in those unable to maintain an upright posture for 30 minutes after taking the medications.

Rarely, biphosphonates have been associated with osteonecrosis of the jaw. Emerging data also suggest that long-term use (>5 years) may lead to fragility fractures, particularly subtrochanteric femur fractures.

Other therapies that may play a role in osteoporosis prevention and treatment include:

- Teriparatide (daily subcutaneous injection, a form of human parathyroid hormone) is approved for individuals with prior fragility fracture or individuals with very low BMD.
- Calcitonin (typically prescribed as a nasal spray, once daily) may reduce spine fracture risk in older women, but is less effective than other approved treatments; it has analgesic properties in the context of acute vertebral fracture.
- Hormone replacement therapy (estrogen) is approved for osteoporosis prevention; benefits must be weighed carefully against risks (e.g. risk of cardiovascular disease and certain cancers).
- Raloxifene (daily PO, a selective estrogen receptor modulator) is approved for osteoporosis prevention/treatment in postmenopausal women; it is generally considered a second-line therapy.

Denosumab (twice yearly subcutaneous injection) is a monoclonal antibody that targets RANK ligand and inhibits osteoclast formation. It is approved for postmenopausal osteoporosis, but is contraindicated in hypocalcemia, which must be corrected prior to dosing.

Although percutaneous balloon vertebroplasty/kyphoplasty have been proposed as treatments for painful vertebral compression fracture, recent studies have suggested only modest benefit. These invasive procedures are generally reserved for those failing more conservative measures.

Fibromyalgia and other soft tissue syndromes

Fibromyalgia

DEFINITION
Fibromyalgia is a process manifest by chronic pain (constant or migratory), multiple trigger points, and minimal evidence of inflammation on either physical examination or laboratory testing.

EPIDEMIOLOGY AND ETIOLOGY/PATHOGENESIS
The disease is relatively common and is most frequently seen in young and perimenopausal women. No clear etiology has been identified, but there is a suggestion that abnormal central nociceptive processing is associated with a decreased pain threshold.

CLINICAL HISTORY AND PHYSICAL EXAMINATION
The patient classically complains of daily pain (which may be migratory), usually associated with or without morning stiffness and a subjective complaint of joint swelling. Many patients present with joint complaints, but when carefully questioned, are describing periarticular complaints. The complaint is often described as a 'burning' sensation and it is common to report a pain scale of greater than 10 (on a 10-point scale). A minority of patients report symptoms of overt depression or acute situational disturbances. American College of Rheumatology (ACR) classification criteria for fibromyalgia requires the presence of 11 or more trigger points (out of a total of 18 points) (**176**).

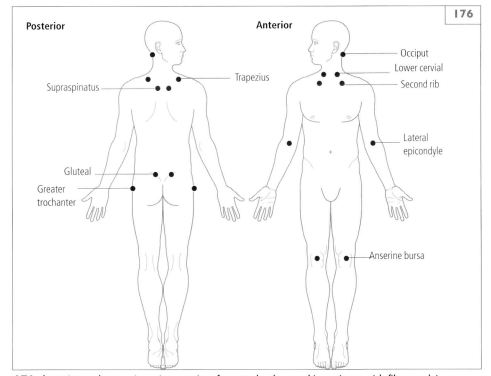

176 Anterior and posterior trigger points frequently observed in patients with fibromyalgia.

DIFFERENTIAL DIAGNOSIS

Chronic pain is a fairly common complaint with a wide differential. In fibromyalgia, there may be an overlap with other causes of chronic pain such as regional pain syndrome, chronic pelvic pain, chronic fatigue syndrome, and other processes such as tension headache. Fibromyalgia may also be seen in patients with concomitant inflammatory or connective tissue diseases including Sjögren's syndrome, lupus, and RA. Secondary causes for diffuse pain, including poor sleep and depression, should be sought (see below). In older patients presenting with bilateral myalgias in a limb-girdle distribution, consideration should be given to the possibility of polymyalgia rheumatica.

INVESTIGATIONS

Fatigue and sleep disturbance are common complaints. Diseases including depression, obstructive sleep apnea, chronic fatigue syndrome, and underlying connective tissue diseases (CTDs), among others, need to be considered.

Laboratory evaluation is characterized by the lack of indicators of inflammation (normal erythrocyte sedimentation rate [ESR] and C-reactive protein [CRP]). Hypothyroidism and sleep disturbances (obstructive sleep apnea, restless leg syndrome, nocturia) can present with fibromyalgia-like complaints and should be considered in the workup. A good rheumatic disease history and physical examination should readily confirm the appropriate diagnosis and obviate the need for more extensive evaluation. Serological and immunological tests are typically normal and usually not necessary for routine evaluation. Radiographic evaluation is not usually necessary and is noncontributory if fibromyalgia is the diagnosis.

PROGNOSIS AND MANAGEMENT

Total alleviation of the symptom complex is usually not obtainable. The patient should be reassured that a serious life-threatening process is not likely. Aerobic exercise is the standard form of management (at least 45 minutes 5 days per week). Behavioral modification (dealing with the chronic pain) may also be necessary. Pharmacologic management is rarely successful on its own. Narcotic analgesics have essentially no role in the treatment of fibromyalgia. Nonsteroidal drugs are relatively nonhelpful. Low-dose tricyclic antidepressants, duloxetine, milnacipran, gabapentin, and pregabalin may be helpful in the treatment of chronic non-nocioreceptive pain. In addition to treatment for comorbid depression (if present), it is essential to identify potential barriers to quality sleep including obstructive sleep apnea and restless leg syndrome.

Regional pain syndromes

Low back and neck pain

Low back and neck pain are common complaints which may be associated with nonspecific musculoskeletal injuries. The physician should be aware that in 95% of individuals with complaints of back and neck pain a muscular etiology exists. Careful history and physical examination are necessary to rule out neurological or skeletal pathology to explain the patient's complaints. 'Red flags' for lower back pain are presented in *Table 61*. Neck pain is most often caused by muscular tension and/or spasm in the shoulders and cervical spine; however, malignancy, infection, trauma, and neurologic etiologies should all be considered in the neck pain differential. In the evaluation of acute neck pain it is important to consider life-threatening conditions such as cardiac angina and carotid dissection. Red flags for neck pain are listed in *Table 62*.

Sciatica describes generally unilateral pain felt in the lower back, buttock, and/or leg and foot which may be accompanied by numbness, weakness, and/or paresthesias. Sciatica is often caused by the compression of the lumbar (L4 or L5) or sacral (S1, S2, or S3) nerve roots, or infrequently by compression of the sciatic nerve. When sciatica is caused by nerve root compression it is considered a lumbar radiculopathy which may be caused by spinal stenosis or a herniated intervertebral disc. Sciatica often resolves with conservative therapy even if a structural abnormality exists. There is no role for oral corticosteroids in the treatment of sciatica.

The majority of patients with neck and back pain will not benefit from radiologic imaging. However, if red flags are present, imaging should generally start with plain radiographs to rule out bone pathology followed by CT or MRI, if indicated, to look for a specific etiology of the patient's complaints. Notably, structural abnormalities, if found, may not correlate with a patient's symptoms. Electromyography (EMG) and nerve conduction velocity (NCV) may be useful when evaluating for neurological compromise.

Table 61 'Red flags' or warning signs for serious underlying pathology in patients presenting with lower back pain

Possible etiologies of low back pain				
Malignancy	**Infection**	**Neurological**	**Abdominal aortic aneurysm**	**Fracture**
History of malignancy	Persistent fever (>100.4°F/38°C)	Saddle anesthesia	Pulsating abdominal mass	Osteoporosis
Unexplained weight loss >10 kg in 6 months	History of IV drug abuse	Urinary incontinence or retention	Atherosclerotic vascular disease	Prolonged use of corticosteroid
Age >50 years	Recent bacterial infection	Decreased anal sphincter tone or incontinence	Age >60 years	Age >70 years
Pain at night or at rest	Immunocompromised state*	Lower extremity weakness or numbness	Pain at night or at rest	Mild trauma over age 50 years
Pain persists for >4–6 weeks		Foot drop		Significant trauma at any age
Failure to improve with treatment		Progressive neurological deficit		

*May include systemic corticosteroids, organ transplant, human immunodeficiency virus, diabetes mellitus, etc.

Key points regarding the management of low back and neck pain include:

- Course is typically self-limited regardless of therapy; recurrences may occur.
- First-line therapy is typically conservative – local heat/ice, acetaminophen, or oral or topical nonsteroidal anti-inflammatory drugs (NSAIDs); a short course of muscle relaxant is used with muscle spasm.
- In carefully selected cases with severe pain, narcotics may be indicated.
- Manual therapies (osteopathic/ chiropractic manipulation) may shorten symptom duration of symptoms and have similar efficacy to NSAIDs.
- For most patients, exercise/physical therapy are critical, and may lessen the severity and frequency of low back pain; in contrast, prolonged bed rest should be discouraged; strengthening of core muscles (through yoga/Pilates) may be particularly beneficial.

Table 62 'Red flags' or warning signs for serious underlying etiologies for neck pain

Preceding accident/injury

Persistent numbness in shoulder or arms

Persistent paresthesias

Weakness

Persistent fever (>100.4°F/38°C)

Persistent sharp shooting pain

Persistent lymph node swelling

Difficulty swallowing

Dizziness/lightheadedness

Other systemic symptoms (i.e. nausea, vomiting)

- Spinal epidural injections may be beneficial in the treatment of radicular symptoms with short-term benefits.
- There is a limited role for surgical therapy, reserved for those with neurological deficits or other pathologic causes (e.g. abdominal aortic aneurysm, tumor); careful patient selection is critical to success.

Complex regional pain syndrome

Complex regional pain syndrome is a condition with unique findings in an extremity usually following a relatively minor proximal event. The patient subsequently develops disabling distal pain, swollen extremity, and vasomotor instability (autonomic dysfunction) which may ultimately result in atrophy of the skin/extremity associated with decreased range of motion. The extremity is usually swollen, cool to the touch (although it may be hyperemic early in the disease process), and quite painful to the touch (**177**). Concomitant radiographs may show significant osteoporosis. Radionuclide imaging can show increased blood flow to the involved joints (**178**). The findings differ from fibromyalgia by the self-limited nature of the complaints (usually only one extremity) and the lack of specific trigger points. Treatment is aggressive physical therapy. Nonsteroidal and other pain medications as well as sympatholytics may have a place in the treatment program.

Nerve entrapment syndromes

Nerve entrapment is common, particularly median nerve compression at the wrist (**179–181**). Patients with carpal tunnel syndrome complain of numbness/pain in their hand but may not describe a classic median nerve distribution. Pain while driving a car (elevation of hands on the steering wheel for some length of time) or awakening at night and having to 'shake' the hand to wake it up are frequently described. Tinel's and Phalen's signs may be demonstrated (**179, 180**). Severe prolonged compression may result in thenar and hypothenar muscle atrophy requiring prompt surgical repair (**181**). Many diverse processes may result in carpal tunnel syndrome. Evaluation for conditions such as pregnancy, hypothyroidism, obesity, RA, and trauma among others should be pursued. In pregnancy, symptoms often abate following delivery. Otherwise, treatment of the underlying entity is required. Evaluation can be done with NCV

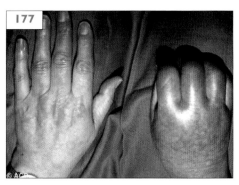

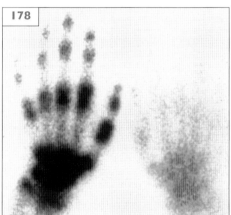

177, 178 A patient with complex regional pain syndrome with involvement of the hand. **177** Diffuse swelling and skin color changes in the right hand; **178:** radionuclide imaging show asymmetric increase in perfusion to the involved hand. (With permission, American College of Rheumatology.)

studies or ultrasound, when median nerve circumference at the level of the pisiform of >10 mm^2 is abnormal (**182**). Steroid injection into the carpal tunnel may be helpful, but surgical release may ultimately be necessary. Ulnar nerve compression, tarsal tunnel syndrome, and Morton's neuroma are examples of other entrapment syndromes that are commonly seen.

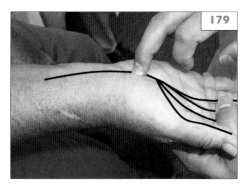

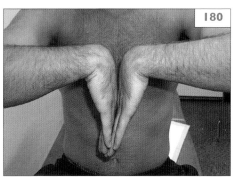

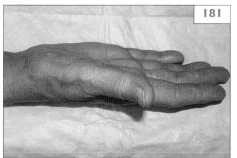

179–181 Carpal tunnel syndrome (CTS). 179: Compression or tapping of the median nerve may elicit numbness in a median nerve distribution (Tinel's sign; 180: symptoms may also be elicited with wrist flexion (positive Phalen's test); 181: longstanding CTS may result in wasting of the thenar eminence. (Courtesy of Dr GF Moore.)

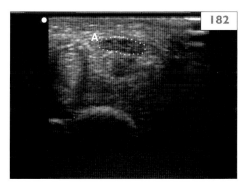

182 Carpal tunnel syndrome; ultrasound image of the median nerve in cross-section shows enlargement of the median nerve (A) with a cross-sectional area of 15 mm^2. A normal median nerve has a cross-sectional area up to 10 mm^2. (Courtesy of Dr AC Cannella.)

Tendinitis/bursitis

Localized musculoskeletal complaints should raise the possibility of periarticular processes such as tendinitis and bursitis. Pain, swelling, and other signs of inflammation are frequently found (**183–185**). A thorough knowledge of anatomy should help with the differential diagnosis. Tenderness over the bicipital groove suggests bicipital tendinitis. Pain with palpation of the lateral epicondyle of the elbow is found in lateral epicondylitis. Olecranon bursitis causes swelling of the olecranon process. Consideration of a septic bursitis should always be kept in mind. Rheumatoid nodules and gouty tophi are commonly found on the extensor surface of the elbows and should be considered when evaluating the patient. Tenderness over the sacroiliac joint may be found in seronegative spondyloarthropathies with sacroiliitis, but can also be one of the trigger points of fibromyalgia. Pain on the lateral aspect of the hip is usually trochanteric bursitis (**184**). These patients will often complain of an inability to sleep on the affected side. True hip pain is in the groin. A common cause of knee pain is osteoarthritis (OA), but tenderness over the inferior medial area of the knee is associated with anserine bursitis (**185**). The anserine bursa is located ~3 cm below the joint margin.

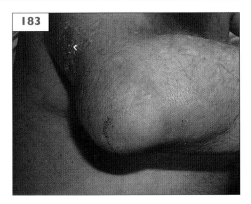

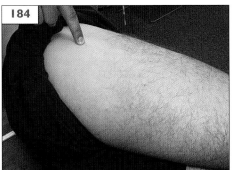

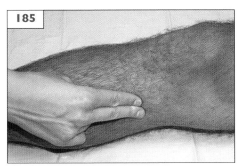

183 Tenderness and swelling over the olecranon bursa in a patient with olecranon bursitis. **184, 185** Tenderness over the greater trochanter (**184**) and anserine bursa (**185**) is indicative of bursitis. (Courtesy of Dr GF Moore.)

Sarcoidosis

DEFINITION
Sarcoidosis is a systemic inflammatory disorder of unknown etiology, characterized by the presence of noncaseating granulomas, and which may manifest with involvement of nearly any organ system, although pulmonary, skin, and ocular involvement is most common.

EPIDEMIOLOGY AND ETIOLOGY
Though sarcoidosis may affect individuals of any age, young adults (ages 20–40 years) are most commonly affected. Women are affected slightly more frequently than are men and significant ethnic and geographic variations in disease prevalence exist. The highest prevalence rates are seen in Sweden, Denmark, and among African-Americans in the US. The natural history of sarcoidosis also varies among racial/ethnic groups. Caucasians are more likely to have erythema nodosum, are less likely to have extrapulmonary manifestations, and have lower age-adjusted mortality. African-Americans tend to have the most severe disease and have the highest mortality. Cardiac and ocular involvement is seen in highest rates in Japanese patients.

The etiology of sarcoidosis is incompletely understood. It has been hypothesized that an environmental exposure with antigenic properties induces an 'aberrant' inflammatory response in a susceptible host. Several potential infectious triggers have been proposed, including mycobacteria, propionobacter species, select viruses (HSV and HHV), and others, though none have been proven. The potential role of environmental exposures in sarcoidosis is supported by observations of disease clustering in nurses, military personnel, and firefighters.

PATHOGENESIS
Sarcoidosis is a disease mediated by CD4+ T cells. Antigen-presenting cells activate T cells resulting in production of proinflammatory cytokines (interleuking [IL]-2, IL-15, interferon [IFN]-γ, and others). CD4+ T cells accumulate within tissues and organize into granulomas.

CLINICAL HISTORY AND PHYSICAL EXAMINATION
As previously mentioned, sarcoidosis can affect nearly any organ system:

- Pulmonary: the most common site of involvement (up to 95%); manifestations include asymptomatic hilar adenopathy (**186**), interstitial lung disease with alveolitis, and endobronchial inflammation resulting in stenosis; it may present with dry cough, dyspnea, or chest pain.
- Ophthalmologic (25–50%): acute anterior uveitis is the most common ocular lesion, often bilateral presenting with blurred vision, photophobia, and increased lacrimation.
- Dermatologic:
  - Erythema nodosum is seen in acute presentations (associated with a benign, self-limited disease course).
  - Lupus presents with a pernio-indurated/violaceous lesion occurring on nose, cheeks, lips, ears, and fingers; slowly progressive; can be disfiguring; associated with pulmonary/osseous involvement.

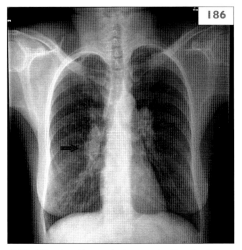

186 Chest radiograph demonstrating the hilar lymphadenopathy typical of sarcoidosis (arrows). (Courtesy of Dr GF Moore.)

- Annular lesions – associated with chronic disease.
- Scars and tattoos can become infiltrated with granulomatous infiltration in patients with sarcoidosis.
- Cardiovascular (rare): May include conduction disturbances, infiltrative cardiomyopathies, papillary muscle dysfunction, sudden cardiac death, congestive heart failure, and pericardial disease.
- Neurological (5%): Central nervous system (CNS) sarcoidosis occurs with predilection for the brainstem and midbrain. Unilateral cranial nerve palsies are most common; a wide variety of neurological manifestations are described.
- Musculoskeletal:
  - Bony involvement (5%): most often asymptomatic, cystic/'lacy' appearance; proximal and middle phalanges are the most common sites (**184**), other sites are less frequent.
  - Acute arthritis: may occur in isolation or as part of Lofgren's syndrome (triad of arthritis, hilar adenopathy, and erythema nodosum); generally involves knees and ankles (mimics reactive arthritis); may have small joint distribution similar to RA or a migratory polyarthritis mimicking rheumatic fever.
  - Muscle involvement: often asymptomatic but may result in weakness due to inflammatory myopathy; three patterns of myopathy are described including: 1) insidious onset of proximal muscle weakness; 2) granulomatous myositis; and 3) nodular myopathy.
  - Osteoporosis/osteopenia: multifactorial owing to glucocorticoids, diffuse skeletal granulomatosis, and increased osteoclastic activity.

DIFFERENTIAL DIAGNOSIS

The differential diagnosis for sarcoidosis is guided by the patient's presenting symptoms. Other systemic, autoimmune disorders such as reactive arthritis (and other spondyloarthritides), RA, systemic lupus erythematosus (SLE), acute rheumatic fever, and others need to be ruled out.

In interpreting results from characteristic tissue biopsy, it is essential that other causes of granulomatous disease including fungal and mycobacterial infection are considered.

INVESTIGATIONS

No laboratory test is diagnostic for sarcoidosis, and most laboratory investigations are aimed at ruling out other differential considerations. A CBC, urinalysis, creatine kinase, and tuberculin skin test are recommended at initial evaluation. Serum angiotensin-converting enzyme (ACE) levels are elevated in 15% of patients with Lofgren's syndrome, but are not diagnostic of, nor useful in screening for sarcoidosis. However, in patients presenting with an acute arthropathy, ACE levels may be prognostically useful. Serum and urinary calcium levels may be elevated in sarcoidosis, but are nonspecific. 1,25-OH vitamin D levels may also be increased due to increased conversion of 25-OH-D by granulomas. A chest X-ray may show bilateral hilar adenopathy or interstitial infiltrates, and high-resolution CT may be useful in further investigating pulmonary involvement, especially in early disease. Bronchiolar lavage will demonstrate an elevated lymphocyte count with predominance of CD4+ T cells. Diagnostic criteria have been established to aid in the identification of sarcoidosis (*Table 63*).

Electrocardiography and pulmonary function testing are recommended in patients diagnosed with sarcoidosis. All patients should have an ophthalmologic evaluation at diagnosis. MRI and positron emission tomography (PET) scans are used primarily to evaluate for involvement of the CNS and heart.

HISTOLOGY

Biopsy of affected organs will typically show well-formed, noncaseating granulomas (**187**). It is important to note that granulomas will not be demonstrated in biopsies of erythema nodosum lesions, and, thus, biopsy of other involved organs may be necessary for diagnosis.

PROGNOSIS

The natural history of sarcoidosis is extremely variable. The majority of patients experience spontaneous remission. Those presenting with acute arthropathy or Lofgren's syndrome typically have a self-limited disease course, though a persistent course is seen in some. Factors associated with a worse prognosis include: multiorgan involvement at presentation, older age at diagnosis, African-American race, duration of illness greater than 6 months, splenomegaly, and lupus pernio.

MANAGEMENT

Sarcoid is usually treated with observation alone, initially. GCs are the mainstay of treatment, and should be used when there is involvement of vital organs (heart, lungs, eyes, CNS). GCs suppress granuloma formation and inhibit fibrosis in sarcoidosis. Immunosuppressive agents are indicated with GC failure or in those who cannot tolerate the side-effects of steroids. Methotrexate (MTX) at doses of 7.5–15 mg per week is the favored treatment in these situations. Azathioprine (AZA) is also effective as a steroid-sparing agent and hydroxychloroquine (HCQ) is effective in the management of cutaneous manifestations and for hypercalcemia/hypercalciuria. Cyclophosphamide (CTX) should be reserved for life-threatening cardiac or neurological manifestations. Infliximab (a monoclonal antibody targeting tumor necrosis factor [TNF]) has been used with success in select patients, mostly those with severe disease.

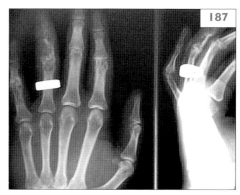

187 Radiographs of the hand showing multiple cystic changes of the proximal and middle phalanges, with destruction of fourth distal interphalangeal joint and narrowing of the second to fifth proximal interphalangeal joints; note the reticular 'lacy' appearance of involved bone. (Courtesy of Dr GF Moore.)

Table 63 Diagnostic criteria for sarcoidosis (WASOG Criteria)

Presence of clinical radiographic features consistent with sarcoidosis

Noncaseating granulomas in one or more organs

Exclusion of other conditions which may mimic sarcoidosis (infections, inhalations, autoimmune disorders)

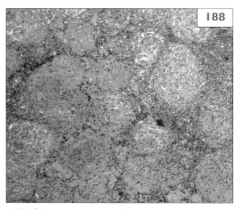

188 Photomicrograph demonstrating multiple noncaseating granulomas typical of biopsied tissue from a patient with sarcoidosis. (Courtesy of Dr GF Moore.)

Amyloidosis

DEFINITION
Amyloidosis is a collection of diseases produced by extracellular deposition of insoluble fibrillar proteins in tissues and organs, and is characterized by systemic multisystem involvement leading to organ failure and death if not treated.

Systemic amyloidosis is classified into four main categories:
- Primary amyloidosis (AL-type).
- Secondary amyloidosis (AA-type).
- Dialysis-related ($A\beta_2M$).
- Familial (ATTR).

EPIDEMIOLOGY AND ETIOLOGY
Amyloidosis incidence increases with age and is rare before age 40 years with similar frequency in men and women. The AL (immunoglobulin light chain)-type is most common. Amyloid-associated (AA)-type amyloidosis occurs in <1% of patients with chronic inflammatory disease (including RA and juvenile idiopathic arthritis; chronic infections including tuberculosis, leprosy, osteomyelitis, and chronic pyleonephritis). Due to a strong association with familial Mediterranean fever (FMF), AA-type amyloidosis is more common in Turkey and the Middle East. AA-type amyloidosis is the only type of amyloidosis to occur in children. Dialysis-related amyloidosis occurs in half of individuals on dialysis for over 12 years and is nearly universal after 15 years of dialysis. Familial amyloidosis overlaps clinically with AL-type amyloidosis and is most often caused by the replacement of valine by methionine at position 30 (Val30Met mutation) in transthyretin (TTR or prealbumin), which produces variant/mutated TTR in the liver. Within families, symptoms tend to occur at about the same age.

PATHOGENESIS
The pathogenesis of each type of amyloidosis is unique; however, they all share the basic process of protein misfolding with subsequent formation of amyloid fibrils. The mechanism by which protein misfolding occurs is currently unknown. AL amyloidosis represents a plasma cell dyscrasia with excess immunoglobulin (Ig) G, IgA, or less commonly, IgM clonal plasma cells in the bone marrow. AL-type amyloidosis can occur in isolation or with multiple myeloma. AA amyloidosis results from deposition of serum amyloid A (SAA). SAA is an acute phase protein which is synthesized in the liver. Amyloid A protein may be produced locally in rheumatoid synovium and SAA levels have been shown to increase with disease activity similar to ESR and CRP. Dialysis-related amyloidosis is generally seen only in patients on long-term hemodialysis with a lower risk for $A\beta_2M$ amyloidosis in peritoneal dialysis patients. Leading theories as to why amyloidosis occurs in long-term dialysis patients include the β_2-microglobulin molecule being too large to pass through a dialysis membrane, as well as the thought that dialysis membranes are bioincompatible and induce proinflammatory mediators which stimulate β_2-microglobulin. Of note, $A\beta_2M$ amyloidosis has rarely been reported in patients with renal failure before dialysis. Familial amyloidosis is due to tissue deposition of mutated TTR which is produced in the liver.

CLINICAL HISTORY AND PHYSICAL EXAMINATION
Disease manifestations are largely determined by type and location of amyloid protein deposits with substantial overlap between the various amyloid types (*Table 64, 189–192 overleaf*).

DIFFERENTIAL DIAGNOSIS
Rheumatic diseases such as RA, lupus, scleroderma (SSc), or spondyloarthopathy may both mimic and co-exist with amyloidosis. It is important to keep a high index of suspicion for amyloidosis in RA patients (or patients with other longstanding systemic inflammatory disease) developing proteinuria.

Table 64 Primary disease manifestations in systemic amyloidosis

AL-type

Fatigue and weight loss (most common)

Carpal tunnel syndrome (positive Tinel sign)

Arthropathy with 'shoulder pad sign' (**189**); other joints include hips, knees, proximal interphalangeal
  joints, distal interphalangeal joints, metacarpal joints, wrists, elbows, and spine

Renal dysfunction with proteinuria, edema, and hypoalbuminemia

Peripheral sensory and motor neuropathy in the lower extremities which progresses to the upper extremities,
  or as autonomic dysfunction (e.g. orthostatic hypotension or abnormal gastrointestinal dysmotility)

Macroglossia (pathognomonic for AL-type) (**190**)

Other organ involvement: purpura, hemorrhagic diathesis, arthropathy, restrictive cardiomyopathy, hepatomegally
  with cholestatic liver disease, functional hyposplenism, xerostomia, muscle pseudohypertrophy, alopecia,
  nail dystrophy, and submandibular gland enlargement

AA-type

Proteinuria and renal insufficiency

Hepatosplenomegally

Autonomic neuropathy

Cardiomyopathy (rare)

Aβ_2M-type (dialysis-associated)

Carpal tunnel syndrome

Persistent joint effusions (large joints such as the shoulder)

Cystic bone lesions (leading to pathologic fractures) (**191, 192**)

Spondyloarthropathy

Familial-type

Microalbuminuria (may be progressive)

Peripheral and/or autonomic neuropathy

Anemia with low erythropoietin levels

Restrictive, nonischemic cardiomyopathy

Vitreous opacities (pathognomic for familial-type)

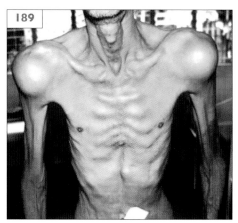

189 'Shoulder pad sign' in a patient with AL-type amyloidosis due to amyloid deposition in periarticular soft tissues. (With permission, New England Journal of Medicine.)

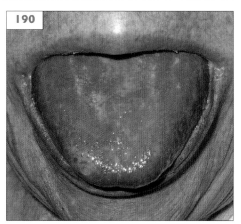

190 Macroglossia in AL-type amyloidosis. (Courtesy of Dr GF Moore.)

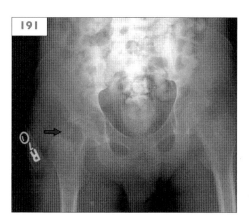

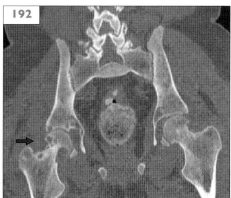

191, 192 Cystic bone lesions which may be seen in $A\beta_2M$-type (dialysis-associated) amyloidosis, most prominent in the right femoral neck. (Courtesy of Dr GF Moore.)

INVESTIGATIONS

Diagnosis is achieved through tissue biopsy demonstrating apple-green birefringence of deposits on polarization microscopy after staining with Congo red (193). Abdominal fat aspirate is the biopsy site of choice as it is minimally invasive with overall positive yield of 60–90% depending on the type of amyloid fibril. If an abdominal fat aspirate is negative and high suspicion of amyloidosis remains, biopsy of a clinically involved organ is appropriate. As treatment differs between types, it is important to differentiate between types of amyloidosis once a tissue diagnosis is confirmed. Additional testing to determine amyloid fibril type through immunofluorescence, immunoperoxidase, and/or immunoelectron microscopy methods should be done after identification of amyloid deposits. With AL-type amyloid, both serum and urine immune fixation electrophoresis (IFE) should be performed together as they are ≥90% sensitive for detection of monoclonal free light chains (FLCs). Detection and quantification of monoclonal FLCs by nephelometry may be complementary to IFE as it allows detection and quantification of FLCs in patients who have no detectable serum or urine M-spike. The sensitivity of serum protein electrophoresis (SPEP) and urine protein electrophoresis (UPEP) are inadequate for diagnosis as the amount of protein may be too low to be quantified.

Additional laboratory evaluations in amyloidosis include monitoring of renal function and urinalysis to evaluate for proteinuria. SAA levels may be elevated in a variety of inflammatory disease as it is a marker of inflammation; however, SAA levels do not correlate with clinical disease. Additional organ-specific testing such as echocardiogram, electrocardiogram, and NCV testing may be necessary depending on clinical manifestations of disease. Joint aspiration demonstrates a noninflammatory synovial fluid and may contain amyloid fibrils.

Radiologic studies (particularly in the dialysis-associated type) may demonstrate a destructive arthritis with findings inclusive of erosions, irregularly shaped hyperlucencies, and subchondral cysts. Ultrasound may demonstrate soft-tissue changes, joint effusions, hyperlucencies, and increased tendon thickness.

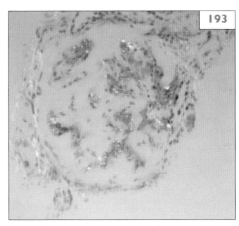

193 Glomerulus stained with Congo red viewed under polarized light microscopy (×400). (Courtesy of Kirk W Foster, MD.)

HISTOLOGY
The primary histological finding in involved tissues in systemic amyloidosis is the presence of apple-green birefringence of deposits under polarized microscopy (**190**).

PROGNOSIS
AL-type amyloidosis is rapidly progressive with a short survival, leading to death on average within 1–1.5 years if untreated. Prognosis is good for AA-type amyloidosis related to chronic inflammatory diseases, with survival usually more than 10 years; however, survival may be significantly limited by renal disease. Prognosis for familial amyloidosis varies by the extent of end-organ involvement. Liver transplant retards the progression of ATTR-type amyloidosis and may improve neuropathy; however, cardiomyopathy and anemia do not improve and may worsen. The course of dialysis-related amyloidosis is generally mild, but a long duration of dialysis and advanced patient age may adversely impact prognosis. Renal transplant may halt progression of $A\beta_2M$-type amyloidosis with disease regression rare.

MANAGEMENT
Treatment of amyloidosis is aimed at reducing the 'supply' of fibril precursors. This is accomplished primarily by treating the underlying inflammation, infection, or malignancy and by elimination of variant proteins.

AL-type amyloidosis is treated similarly to multiple myeloma with high-dose melphalan combined with autologous stem cell transplant being the most effective therapy (5-year survival rate >50%). As transplantation-related mortality rates may be as high as 25%, oral melphalan and corticosteroids, though rarely eliminating the plasma cell dyscrasia, may be used (5-year survival rate 36%). Other options for AL-type amyloidosis with less available data include thalidomide, lenalidomide, and proteasome inhibitors.

AA-type amyloidosis is treated by addressing the underlying inflammatory disorder or infection. For FMF-related AA amyloidosis, colchicine 1.2–1.8 mg/day is the treatment of choice; however, colchicine is not effective for other causes of amyloidosis.

In dialysis-related amyloidosis, renal transplant normalizes plasma levels of β_2-microglobulin with subsequent slow decreases in tissue amyloid deposits. Improvements in dialysis equipment and techniques (i.e. copper-free dialysis membranes) appear to be useful in decreasing disease frequency and symptoms.

For ATTR-type amyloidosis, orthotopic liver transplant is the treatment of choice. Liver transplant removes the major source of variant TTR production and replaces it with normal TTR. Diflunisal, a salicylate drug with NSAID activity has been shown to stabilize variant TTR in clinical trials.

Supportive treatment (i.e. nutritional support, dialysis, organ transplant, cardiac pacemaker) for specific disease manifestations should be offered to patients with all types of amyloidosis. Due to avid binding to cardiac amyloid which produces unpredictable pharmacokinetics, digitalis, calcium channel blockers, and beta-blockers are relatively contraindicated in patients with amyloidosis.

Miscellaneous rheumatic conditions

AVASCULAR NECROSIS OR OSTEONECROSIS

Avascular necrosis (AVN) or osteonecrosis (also known as aseptic necrosis, ischemic necrosis, and osteochondritis dissecans) are terms used to describe cellular death in bone, resulting from a loss of blood supply which leads to the loss of bone integrity and, in severe cases, marked destruction of bony architecture (**194, 195**). AVN may be classified as: primary (idiopathic) *vs.* secondary (related to a known risk factor, e.g. GC use) or traumatic *vs.* nontraumatic. Conditions and other risk factors for AVN are summarized in *Table 65*.

AVN most commonly involves the femoral head, less often occurring in the humeral head, femoral condyles (knee), tibial plateau, or small bones of the hands/feet. Multifocal involvement may occur. Osteonecrosis of the jaw (ONJ) has been described as a recent complication of bisphosphonate therapy, typically in the context of underlying malignancy. The pathogenesis of AVN, although not completely understood, involves ischemic injury, typically related to disruption of blood supply. Although rarely asymptomatic, patients with AVN typically present with pain including deep groin pain in patients with hip involvement. AVN is most often diagnosed using radiographs, but may require MRI or three-phase bone scan early in the disease process when radiographs may be falsely normal. Treatment is typically conservative (bed rest, reduced weight bearing) with judicious analgesia/NSAIDs. Although once popular, surgical core decompression is rarely indicated in the treatment of AVN.

BASIC CALCIUM PHOSPHATE AND CALCIUM OXALATE CRYSTAL DEPOSITION

In addition to the deposition of monosodium urate (MSU, causing gout) and calcium pyrophosphate (CPPD, causing pseudogout) crystals, basic calcium phosphate (BCP) crystal deposition can occur, resulting in an inflammatory arthritis and/or periarthritis.

Hydroxyapatite (HA) crystals are the most common form of BCP. In contrast to MSU and CPPD crystals, HA and other forms of BCP are not readily identifiable under polarized microscopy given their small size. BCP aggregates can occasionally be visualized as 'shiny coins' under light microscopy, and Alizarin red S stain (which binds to calcium) has been suggested as a 'screen' for the presence of BCP crystals. BCP deposition has been associated with a variety of clinical presentations including calcific periarthritis (including gout-like pseudopodagra) and Milwaukee shoulder syndrome (MSS). MSS is more common in women (80% of cases) and is associated with a marked rotator cuff tendonopathy leading to pain and dysfunction. Radiographically, MSS is associated with degenerative changes in the glenohumeral

194 Shoulder radiograph in a patient with lupus and long-term prednisone use; subcortical bone collapse in the superiomedial aspect of the left humeral head, consistent with avascular necrosis (arrows). (Courtesy of Dr GF Moore.)

Table 65 Conditions/risk factors associated with avascular necrosis

Glucocorticoid use

Trauma – fractures

Coagulopathy – e.g. antiphospholipid antibody syndrome, myeloproliferative disease, sickle cell, etc.

Radiation therapy

Gaucher disease

Toxins – alcohol

Inflammatory/autoimmune diseases – lupus, rheumatoid arthritis, inflammatory bowel disease

Bisphosphonate use in malignancy

Embolism/fat necrosis/decompression disease (caisson disease)

Pregnancy

Solid organ transplantation

Human immunodeficiency virus

195 Pelvic radiograph showing loss of bony architecture in both femoral heads (flattening) in a patient with longstanding prednisone use, consistent with avascular necrosis. (Courtesy of Dr GF Moore.)

joint, the presence of soft tissue calcifications, and a 'high riding' humeral head (**196**). Synovial fluid analyses in MSS typically reveal high red blood cell counts and low leukocyte counts. BCP aggregates (shiny coins) may be visualized and Alizarin red S stain may be positive. Often treatment refractory, NSAIDs and repeated aspirations are often used. Total shoulder replacement may be indicated for pain relief in the context of severe degenerative disease when other treatment measures have failed.

Inflammatory arthritis rarely occurs secondary to calcium oxalate deposition, either from primary oxylosis or the secondary oxalosis seen in chronic dialysis patients. Clinical presentations often mimic those seen in gout or pseudogout, although end-organ involvement has been described with calcium oxalate including peripheral vascular disease and gangrene, cardiac disease, and neuropathy. In the context of renal dialysis, treatment is geared towards prevention with effective dialysis and maintenance of an 'optimal' calcium–phosphorous product.

HEMOCHROMATOSIS, OCHRONOSIS (ALKAPTONURIA), AND WILSON'S DISEASE

Arthritis may occur as a consequence of heritable metabolic disorders including hemochromatosis, ochronosis (alkaptonuria), and Wilson's disease, all with autosomal recessive inheritance. These disorders are all associated with secondary degenerative joint disease, which may be heralded by a joint distribution distinct from primary OA.

Hemochromatosis is characterized by the accumulation of iron in affected tissues, leading clinically to liver disease (cirrhosis), cardiomyopathy, diabetes (due to pancreatic deposition and islet cell failure), skin hyperpigmentation, and elevated serum iron and iron saturation (screening blood tests for hemochromatosis). An iron to iron binding capacity ratio exceeding 50% warrants additional evaluation, with the diagnosis most commonly confirmed through genotyping. Hemochromatosis is associated with degenerative arthropathy in addition to CPPD/chondrocalcinosis. Hands, knees, and hips are the most commonly affected joints. In addition to chondrocalcinosis, characteristic radiographic findings include joint space narrowing, subchondral cysts, and hooked radial osteophytes of the metacarpal–phalangeal (MCP) and proximal interphalangeal (PIP) joints (**197**). Treatment of hemochromatosis includes phlebotomy or iron chelation, which appears to reverse damage due to end-organ iron accumulation. Iron removal, however, does not appear to ameliorate the course of arthritis, for which treatment is often symptomatic with NSAIDs, other analgesics, and exercise.

Ochronosis is a hereditary disorder resulting from a defect in the oxidation of homogentisic acid. As a result of this defect, pigment is deposited and accumulates in cartilage and other connective tissues. Clinically, this abnormal pigment deposition is reflected in pigmentation of the skin and surrounding tissues (pinna of the ear, sclera) and a progressive degenerative arthritis, the latter due to deposition in cartilage and subsequent breakdown. In addition to showing typical findings of degenerative arthritis (leading to spondyloarthropathy or a peripheral arthropathy), spine radiographs may show characteristic calcifications of the intervertebral discs. Synovial fluid is typically noninflammatory while a near pathognomonic 'ground pepper' sign (black ochronotic shards suspended in the synovium) may be seen. For ochronotic-related arthropathy, treatment is typically symptomatic.

Wilson's disease is a heritable (autosomal recessive) disorder of copper metabolism, characterized clinically by the deposition of gold-brown pigment at the corneal margin (the so-called Kayser–Fleischer ring). Similar to hemochromatosis and ochronosis, Wilson's disease is associated with diffuse osteopenia in addition to the development of 'premature' degenerative arthritis with a joint distribution that is atypical for primary OA. The wrist is most commonly affected but may involve other joints including the hands, elbow, shoulder, hip, and knee. Chondrocalcinosis and periarticular calcifications may be seen on radiographs. Synovial fluid is typically noninflammatory and the diagnosis is based on elevations in serum ceruloplasmin. Treatment is focused on copper chelation with D-penicillamine, although it is not yet clear whether chelation therapy alters the long-term course of arthritis in Wilson's disease.

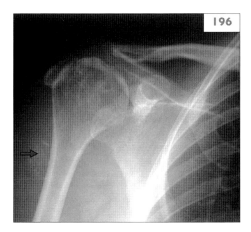

196 Shoulder radiograph in a patient with presumed Milwaukee shoulder syndrome (arthropathy secondary to hydroxyapatite crystal deposition); findings include superior subluxation of humeral head with marked glenohumeral degenerative changes and soft tissue calcifications laterally (arrow).

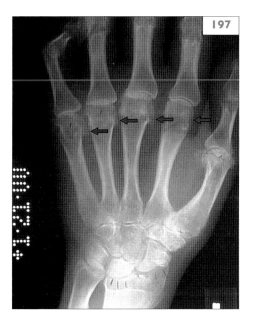

197 Hand radiograph in patient with hemochromatosis, showing marked degenerative changes in metacarpal–phalangeal (MCP) and proximal interphalangeal, and wrist joints. Note radial hooked osteophytes (arrows), most notable on the second and third MCP joints.

HERITABLE DISORDERS OF BONE AND CARTILAGE

Hereditary disorders affecting bone, cartilage, and other connective tissues often have rheumatic manifestations. For example, patients with Ehlers–Danlos (**198, 199**) may present with joint laxity and polyarthralgias while patients with osteogenesis imperfecta (**200, 201**) may present with fracture. Although a comprehensive review of all known heritable disorders affecting bone and cartilage is beyond the scope of this section, entities more commonly encountered in rheumatology practice are summarized in *Table 66*.

HYPERTROPHIC OSTEOARTHROPATHY

Hypertrophic osteoarthropathy (HOA) is a form of arthritis associated with digital clubbing and periostitis with subperiosteal bone formation in long bones. HOA is classified as primary or secondary.

Primary HOA, also known as pachydermo-periostitis, is an autosomal dominant disorder with variable penetrance. Rare, primary HOA is characterized by cylindrical thickening of the extremities in addition to clubbing, excessive sweating, and thickening of facial skin.

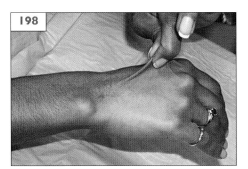

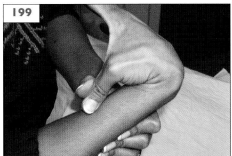

198, 198 Findings in Ehlers–Danlos syndrome (classic type) include increased extensibility of the skin (**195**) and joint laxity (**196**). (Courtesy of Dr GF Moore.)

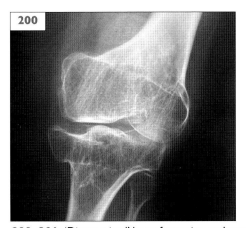

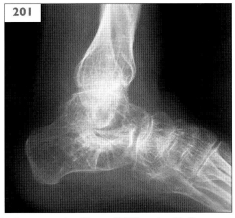

200, 201 'Disorganized' bone formation and marked osteopenia of knee (**200**) and ankle/foot (**201**) on X-ray in a patient with osteogenesis imperfecta, Type I.

Table 66 Select heritable disorders of bone and cartilage with rheumatic manifestations

Disorder	Inheritance	Signs/symptoms
Albright hereditary osteodystrophy	Variable	Short stature; bradydactyly; variable mental redardation; resistance to PTH (increased iPTH; hypocalcemia and hyperphosphatemia)
Ehlers–Danlos syndromes **(198, 199)**	Variable	Several types (I–XI); joint hypermobility with polyarthralgias; laxity in other connective tissues based on type (most commonly skin)
Familial joint hypermobility	Variable	Joint laxity and polyarthralgias; early degenerative disease possible
Homocystinuria	Autosomal recessive	Lens dislocation; arachnodactyly; chest/spinal deformity; osteoporosis; 'tight' joints; vascular thrombosis; malar flushing; psychiatric disease; mental retardation; valvular disease; aortic aneurysm
Marfan syndrome	Autosomal dominant	Marked joint laxity with polyarthralgias; lens dislocation and myopia; unique body habitus (disproportionately long extremities); lens dislocation; arachnodactyly; chest/spinal deformity; valvular disease; aortic aneurysm/valvular disease
Osteogenesis imperfecta **(200, 201)**	Variable/autosomal dominant (Type I) most common	Types I–V; Type I most common: bone fragility and fracture; blue sclera; hearing loss
Stickler syndrome	Autosomal dominant	Myopia/retinal detachment; facial dysmorphia; progressive hearing loss; variable mental retardation; joint laxity with polyarthralgias and early-onset degenerative arthritis

Secondary HOA accompanies other illnesses, most often pulmonary tumors or infections. Conditions assoiated with secondary HOA are shown in *Table 67*. Patients with HOA may be asymptomatic or may have severe disabling bone and joint pain with oligoarthritis or polyarthritis. Examination findings include digital clubbing (**202**) and less often visible widening and warmth over involved bone. While acute phase reactants (e.g. ESR) may be elevated, synovial fluid is typically noninflammatory. Radiographs (or alternatively, nuclear bone scan) characteristically show evidence of new periosteal bone formation in the diaphyseal regions of long bones (**203**). Chest imaging is vital in the evaluation of HOA, particularly in those with a history of smoking (**204**). Although not fully understood, the pathogenesis of HOA appears to involve increased expression of vascular endothelial growth factor (VEGF). Thyroid acropachy is a related disorder characterized by digital clubbing and periostitis, typically in the context of previous or current hyperthyroidism. Management of HOA includes:

- Treatment of underlying conditions (e.g. tumor resection).
- Vagotomy.
- Symptomatic treatment with NSAIDs/other analgesics.
- Bisphosphonates (IV pamidronate).
- GCs.
- Parenteral octreotide.

NEUROPATHIC JOINT DISEASE (CHARCOT JOINTS)

Neuropathic joint disease is a progressive form of degenerative arthritis related to denervation and a loss of protective proprioception. Patients may present with pain and joint swelling, although pain may be minimal in the context of severe neuropathy.

Causes of neuropathic joint disease include:

- Diabetes mellitus complicated by neuropathy (most common); typically involves the forefoot and ankle.
- Syphilis (tabes dorsalis) affecting the knee.
- Syringomyelia affecting the shoulder or elbow.

Characteristic radiographic finding of Charcot joint include marked joint subluxation with malalignment, bony fragmentation, simultaneous areas of bone formation and

Table 67 Conditions associated with secondary HOA

Pulmonary
Bronchogenic carcinoma/pleural tumors
Cystic fibrosis
Chronic bronchitis
Bronchiectasis
Empyema
Interstitial pulmonary fibrosis
Tuberculosis/chronic fungal infections

Cardiac
Congenital heart disease

Gastrointestinal
Inflammatory bowel disease
Biliary atresia

resorption, and the presence of periarticular debris (**205**). Pseudo-Charcot joints have been described in severe forms of CPPD arthropathy, although rare. Treatment of neuropathic joint disease is focused on symptom relief and the prevention of progressive joint destruction (e.g. optimizing diabetic control, bracing, selective nonweight bearing).

PAGET'S DISEASE

Paget's disease of the bone is characterized by dysregulated bone turnover. The prevalence of Paget's disease based on radiographic surveys may be as high as 1–2%, although symptomatic disease is far less common. Paget's likely has a genetic component (based on observations of familial clustering) with speculation that a viral infection (respiratory syncitial virus [RSV], canine distemper virus) could trigger the disease. Although frequently asymptomatic (often found incidentally on imaging studies), signs and symptoms of Paget's disease may include:

- Bone and joint pains; back pain with spinal stenosis; secondary OA.

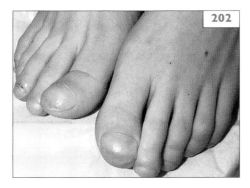

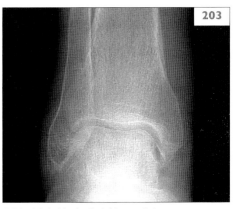

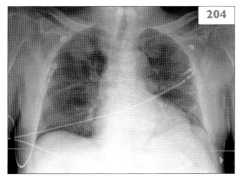

202–204 Marked clubbing of the toes in a patient with cystic fibrosis and secondary hypertrophic osteoarthropathy (**202**). New periosteal bone formation of the distal tibia (most prominent on the medial aspect) in a patient with secondary hypertrophic osteoarthropathy (**203**). Chest X-ray with right apical mass from a patient with secondary hypertrophic osteoarthropathy; subsequent biopsy confirmed a diagnosis of bronchogenic carcinoma (**204**). (Courtesy of Dr GF Moore.)

205 Ankle radiograph in a patient with poorly controlled diabetes mellitus, diabetic neuropathy, and complaints of progressive 'swelling' of the foot and ankle. Radiograph shows marked bony malalignment with sclerosis and bony debris, consistent with neuropathic joint disease (Charcot joint). (Courtesy of Dr GF Moore.)

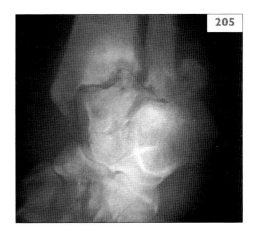

- Malignancy (rare transformation into osteosarcoma).
- High output heart failure (increased vascularity/metabolic demand in bone).
- Hearing loss (petrous bony extension into the cochlea).
- Mental status changes (hydrocephalus).
- Motor loss (spinal cord compression).
- Hypercalcemia (rarely occurs with immobilization).
- Elevations in serum alkaline phosphatase.

The pelvis is involved in a majority of cases with less frequent involvement in the skull, spine, and lower extremity (femur and tibia). Radiographs show marked 'disorganization' with concomitant osteolytic and osteoblastic changes (**206**). Skull involvement may show classic 'cotton wool' lesions. Vertebral involvement may manifest with classic 'ivory spine' due to bony enlargement and increased radiodensity on X-ray. Nuclear bone scan may provide additional sensitivity in detecting areas of new bone formation in Paget's, with intense diffuse uptake in the skull being characteristic. Bisphosphonates (alendronate, risedronate, pamidronate) are the primary treatment modality for Paget's bone disease; serum alkaline phosphatase levels may be helpful in monitoring the effectiveness of treatment.

PIGMENTED VILLONODULAR SYNOVITIS

Pigmented villonodular synovitis (PVNS) is a 'benign' tumor of the joint, most commonly affecting the knee and hip, although other joints can be involved. Patients typically present with progressive joint pain and swelling with recurrent bloody effusions. Synovial aspirates may have a characteristic 'chocolate' color. The tumor can lead to destructive changes (**207**), hemosiderin deposition, and inflammatory changes related to recurrent intra-articular bleeding. Diagnosis of PVNS is confirmed through synovial biopsy (showing visible papillae) and definitive treatment involves surgical synovectomy.

POPLITEAL (BAKER) CYST

Popliteal (Baker) cysts represent posterior protrusions of synovial fluid and synovial tissues in the knee. Popliteal cysts frequently complicate pre-existing knee arthritis, most commonly OA, although they can be seen in forms of inflammatory arthritis (e.g. RA). Popliteal cysts may be asymptomatic or can cause pain or a sensation of knee swelling/tightness, particularly with knee flexion. With extension or rupture of popliteal cysts, the patient may experience acute calf pain and swelling with accompanying erythema or echymosis. A ruptured popliteal cyst can mimic deep venous thrombosis. Popliteal cysts are typically diagnosed based on examination findings (popliteal fullness) and confirmed through appropriate imaging studies (usually ultrasound or MRI) (**208**). Treatment of popliteal cysts includes treating the underlying arthritis in addition to the intra-articular injection of GCs. Rarely, surgical excision of the cyst may be indicated.

MALIGNANCY AND RHEUMATIC DISEASES

There are several known associations between rheumatic disease and malignancy. Malignancy can develop after years of rheumatic disease, such as lymphoma and RA. Some rheumatic diseases can be a manifestation of malignancy (paraneoplastic), such as dermatomyositis. Finally, some of the medications used to treat rheumatic disease can increase the risk of malignancy, such as cyclophosphamide and bladder cancer. The commonly known paraneoplastic syndromes and rheumatic disease and medication-associated malignancies are shown in *Tables 68* and *69 overleaf*

ENDOCRINOPATHIES AND RHEUMATIC MANIFESTATIONS

Musculoskeletal complaints can be very common in disorders of the endocrine system:

- Diabetes mellitus has a variety of joint complications, particularly in the hand. The diabetic stiff hand syndrome (diabetic cheiroarthropathy) resembles SSc in its late stages with thick, shiny and inelastic tissue (**209**). Dupuytren's contractures and trigger fingers are also common (**210**). Other upper extremity findings include adhesive capsulitis, reflex sympathetic dystrophy, and carpal tunnel syndrome. Charcot's arthropathy and osteomyelitis can be seen in the feet, and diffuse idiopathic skeletal hyperostosis is seen in the spine. Diabetic amyopathy also occurs and is manifest by pain and atrophy in large muscle groups.
- Hyperparathyroidism results in osteopenia, chondrocalcinosis, and proximal muscle weakness. When secondary to renal disease, renal osteodystrophy occurs and involves an erosive arthritis of the hands and bony resorption of the distal clavicle.
- Hypoparathyroidism results in proximal muscle weakness.
- Hyperthyroidism results in osteoporosis, proximal muscle weakness, and thyroid acropachy (clubbing and periostitis). Individuals with Grave's disease and Hashimoto's thyroiditis commonly have a positive antinuclear antibody.

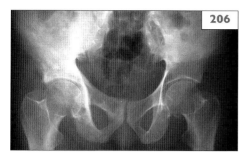

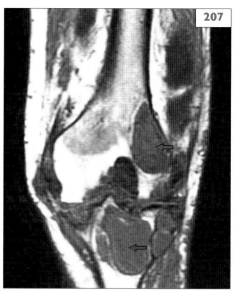

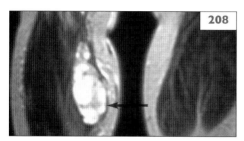

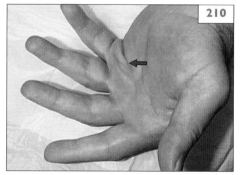

206–208 Pelvic radiograph in a patient with Paget's disease of the bone; note 'disorganized' bone formation with simultaneous areas of sclerosis and lytic changes of the right ileum and pubic ramus (**206**). MRI of knee showing hemosiderin deposition (arrows) and destructive changes in a patient with biopsy confirmed pigmented villonodular synovitis (**207**). (Courtesy of Dr GF Moore.) MRI of knee in patient with osteoarthritis, showing a large popliteal cyst with extension into the calf (right knee, arrow), with marked enhancement on T2-weighted image (white area) (**208**).

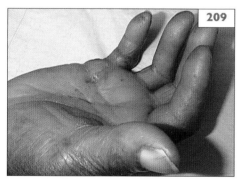

209 Diabetic cheirarthropathy in a patient with poorly controlled type II diabetes mellitus; note skin changes resembling those of scleroderma manifested by thickened, shiny, and inelastic skin. (Courtesy of Dr GF Moore.)

210 Dupuytren's contractures in a patient with poorly controlled diabetes; note fibrotic, palpable flexor tendons over the palm (arrow) with resulting flexion contractures most evident in the fourth and fifth digits. (Courtesy of Dr GF Moore.)

- Hypothyroidism can cause joint swelling, chondrocalcinosis, proximal muscle weakness, and carpal tunnel syndrome.
- Acromegaly (due to increased levels of growth hormone) results in carpal tunnel syndrome, Raynaud's phenomenon, premature osteoarthritis, and back pain.
- Pregnancy results in a variety of musculoskeletal problems, including low back pain, and carpal tunnel syndrome.

Table 68 Paraneoplastic syndromes with rheumatic manifestations

Rheumatic disease	Malignancy
Carcinomatous polyarthritis (seronegative inflammatory arthritis)	Solid tumors (breast, lung, colon, ovarian) Lymphoproliferative disorders
Cutaneous vasculitis	Lymphoproliferative disorders Myeloproliferative disorders
Panniculitis	Breast, pancreatic, and prostate cancer Hematologic malignancies
Fasciitis (palmar with polyarthritis)	Ovarian, breast, gastric, and pancreatic cancers
Complex regional pain syndrome	Pancoast tumor
Erythromelalgia	Hematologic malignancies
Polymyalgia rheumatica	Kidney, lung, and colon cancer Multiple myeloma
Remitting seronegative symmetric synovitis with pitting edema	Lymphoma Myelodysplastic syndrome Adenocarcinoma
Multicentric reticulohistiocytosis	Solid tumors (breast, lung, stomach, cervix, colon, ovary)
Dermatomyositis > polymyositis	Solid tumors (ovarian, lung, gastric)

Table 69 Associations of rheumatic diseases and medications used to treat rheumatic diseases with malignancy

Rheumatic disease	Malignancy
Sjögren's syndrome	Lymphoproliferative disorder
Rheumatoid arthritis	
Progressive systemic sclerosis	Lung and esophageal cancer
Medications	
Cyclophosphamide	Hematologic malignancy, bladder and skin cancer
Azathioprine	Non-Hodgkin's lymphoma
Methotrexate	Lymphoma (Epstein–Barr virus association)
Anti-tumor necrosis factor-α biologic agents	

Further Reading

Chapter 1
Overview of Rheumatology and Rheumatic Conditions

INTRODUCTION

Helmick CG, Felson DT, Lawrence RC, *et al*. (2008). Estimates of the prevalence of arthritis and other rheumatic conditions in the United States. Part I. *Arthritis Rheum* **58**:15–25.

Silman AJ, Hochberg MC (eds) (2001). *Epidemiology of the Rheumatic Diseases*, 2nd edn, Oxford, New York.

SYNOPSIS OF IMMUNOLOGY IN RHEUMATIC DISEASE

Doan T, Melvold R, Viselli S, Waltenbaugh C (eds) (2008). *Lippincott's Illustrated Reviews Immunology*, Lippincott Williams & Wilkins, Philadelphia.

Janeway CA, Travers P, Walport M, Shlomchik MJ (eds) (2005). *Immunobiology: the Immune System in Health and Disease*, 6th edn, Garland Science, London.

Male D, Brostoff J, Roth DB, Roitt I (eds) (2006). *Immunology*, 7th edn, Mosby Elsevier, Philadelphia.

ASSESSMENT OF THE PATIENT WITH A SUSPECTED RHEUMATIC CONDITION

Brower AC (1997). *Arthritis in Black and White*, 2nd edn. Saunders, Philadelphia.

Mikuls TR (2004). Synovial fluid analysis. In: *Arthritis and Allied Health Conditions*, 15th edn. Koopman WJ, Moreland LW (eds). Philadelphia, Williams & Wilkins, pp. 81–96.

Peter JB, Schoenfield Y (eds) (1996). *Autoantibodies*. Elsevier, Philadelphia.

PREGNANCY IN RHEUMATIC DISEASES

Clowse ME (2010). Managing contraception and pregnancy in the rheumatologic diseases. *Best Pract Res Clin Rheumatol* **24**:373–85.

PHARMACOLOGICAL TREATMENT OF RHEUMATIC DISEASE

Cannella AC, O'Dell JR (2002). Cytotoxic, immunoregulatory, and biologic agents. In: *Rheumatology Secrets*, 2nd edn. West SG (ed). Hanley & Belfus, Philadelphia, pp. 588–98.

Morand AF, Goulding NJ (1993). Glucocorticoids in rheumatoid arthritis – mediators and mechanisms. *Br J Rheum* **32**:816–19.

O'Dell JR, Cannella AC (2008). Methotrexate, leflunomide, sulfasalazine, hydroxychloroquine, and combination therapies. In: *Kelley's Textbook of Rheumatology*, 8th edn. Firestein GS, Budd RC, Harris Jr. ED, McInnes IB, Ruddy S, Sergent JS (eds). Saunders Elsevier, Philadelphia, pp. 883–907.

Simon LS (1995). Actions and toxicity of nonsteroidal anti-inflammatory drugs. *Curr Opin Rheum* **7**:159–66.

NONPHARMACOLOGICAL TREATMENT OF RHEUMATIC DISEASE

Ettinger WH Jr, Burns R, Messier SP, *et al*. (1997). A randomized trial comparing aerobic exercise and resistance exercise with a health education program in older adults with knee osteoarthritis. *JAMA* **277**(1):25–31.

Fortin P, Clarke A, Joseph L, *et al*. (1999). Outcomes of total hip and knee replacement: preoperative functional status predicts outcomes at six months after surgery. *Arthritis Rheum* **42**:1722.

Gossec L, Pavy S, Pham T, *et al*. (2006). Nonpharmacological treatments in early rheumatoid arthritis: clinical practice guidelines based on published evidence and expert opinion. *Joint Bone Spine* **73**:396–402.

Chapter 2
Osteoarthritis and Inflammatory Arthritis

OSTEOARTHRITIS

Altman R, Asch E, Bloch D, *et al*. (1986). Development of criteria for the classification and reporting of osteoarthritis: a classification of osteoarthritis of the knee. *Arthritis Rheum* **29**(8):1039–49.

Felson DT, Lawrence RC, Dieppe PA, *et al*. (2000). Osteoarthritis: new insights. Part 1: The disease and its risk factors. *Ann Intern Med* **133**(8):635–46.

Hochberg MC, Altman RD, April KT *et al*. American College of Rheumatology. Recommendations for the use of nonpharmacologic and pharmacologic therapies in osteoarthritis of the hand, hip and knee: *Arthritis Care Res* 2012 **64**:455–74.

RHEUMATOID ARTHRITIS
McInnes IB, O'Dell JR (2010). State-of the-art: rheumatoid arthritis. *An nRheum Dis* **69**:898–906.
Mikuls TR (2003). Co-morbidity in rheumatoid arthritis. *Best Pract Res Clin Rheumatol* **5**:929–52.
Saag KG, Teng GG, Patkar NM, *et al*. (2008). American College of Rheumatology 2008 recommendations for the use of nonbiologic and biologic disease-modifying antirheumatic drugs in rheumatoid arthritis. *Arthritis Rheum* **59**:762–84.
Van der Linden MP, Knevel R, Huizinga TW, van der Helm-van Mil AH (2011). Classification of rheumatoid arthritis: comparison of the 1987 American College of Rheumatology criteria and the 2010 American College of Rheumatology/ European League Against Rheumatism criteria. *Arthritis Rheum* **63**:37–42.

GOUT
Cannella AC, Mikuls TR (2005). Understanding treatments for gout. *Am J Manag Care* **11**(15 Suppl):S451–8.
Terkeltaub R (2010). Update on gout: new therapeutic strategies and options. *Nat Rev Rheumatol* **6**:30–8.
Zhang W, Doherty M, Pascual E, *et al* (2006). EULAR evidence based recommendations for gout. Part I and II: Diagnosis and Management. Report of a task force of the Standing Committee for International Clinical Studies Including Therapeutics (ESCISIT). *Ann Rheum Dis* **65**:1301–11, 1312–24.

CPPD DEPOSITION, PSEUDOGOUT, AND CHRONDROCALCINOSIS
Ryan LM, McCarty DJ (1993). Calcium pyrophosphate crystal deposition disease: pseudogout, articular chondrocalcinosis. In: *Arthritis and Allied Conditions*, 12th edn. McCarty DJ, Koopman WJ (eds). Philadelphia, Lea and Febiger, pp.1835–55.

ADULT-ONSET STILL'S DISEASE
Bagnari V, Colina M, Ciancio G, Govoni M, Trotta F (2010). Adult-onset Still's disease. *Rheumatol Int* **30**:855–62.
Efthimiou P, Paik PK, Bielory L (2006). Diagnosis and management of adult onset Still's disease. *Ann Rheum Dis* **65**:564–72.

SEPTIC ARTHRITIS
Baker DG, Schumacher Jr. HR (1993). Acute monoarthritis [review]. *NEJM* **329**:1013–20.
Goldenberg DL (1998). Septic arthritis. *Lancet* **351**:197–202.
Goldenberg DL, Reed JI (1985). Bacterial arthritis. *NEJM* **312**:764–71.

VIRAL ARTHRITIS
Cacoub P, Poynard T, Ghillani P, *et al*. (1999). Extrahepatic manifestations of chronic hepatitis C. *Arthritis Rheum* **42**:2204-12.
Vassilopoulos D, Calabrese LH (2008). Virally associated arthritis 2008: clinical, epidemiologic, and pathophysiologic considerations. *Arthritis Res Ther* **10**:215.

LYME DISEASE
Steere AC (2001). Medical progress: Lyme disease. *NEJM* **345**:115–25.

RHEUMATIC FEVER
Lee JL, Naguwa SM, Cheema GS, Gershwin ME (2009). Acute rheumatic fever and its consequences: a persistent threat to developing nations in the 21st century. *Autoimmun Rev* **9**:117–23.
Van der Helm-van Mil AH (2010). Acute rheumatic fever and poststreptococcal reactive arthritis reconsidered. *Curr Opin Rheumatol* **22**:437–42.

Chapter 3
Seronegative
Spondyloarthropathy

SPONDYLOARTHROPATHY OVERVIEW
Healy P, Helliwell P (2005). Classification of the spondyloarthropathies. *Curr Opin Rheumatol* **17**:395.
Olivieri I, van Tubergen A, Salvarani C, van der Linden S (2002). Seronegative spondyloarthritides. *Best Pract Res Clin Rheumatol* **16**:723–39.

ANKYLOSING SPONDYLITIS

Brown M, Kennedy G, MacGregor A, *et al*. (1997). Susceptibility to ankylosing spondylitis in twins – the role of genes, HLA, and the environment. *Arthritis Rheum* **49**:1823.

Van den Bosch R, De Keyser F, Mielants H, Veys E (2005). Tumor necrosis factor-alpha blockade in ankylosing spondylitis: a potent but expensive anti-inflammatory treatment or true disease modification? *Arthritis Res Ther* 7:121.

Wanders A, Heijde D, Landewe R, Behier J, *et al*. (2005). Nonsteroidal anti-inflammatory drugs reduce radiographic progression in patients with ankylosing spondylitis: a randomized clinical trial. *Arthritis Rheum* **52**:1756.

REACTIVE ARTHRITIS

Carter JD, Hudson AP (2010). The evolving story of *Chlamydia*-induced reactive arthritis. *Curr Opin Rheumatol* **22**:424–30.

Colmegna I, Espinoza L (2005). Recent advances in reactive arthritis. *Curr Rheumatol Rep* 7:201.

Townes JM, Deodhar AA, Laine ES, *et al*. (2008). Reactive arthritis following culture-confirmed infections with bacterial enteric pathogens in Minnesota and Oregon: a population-based study. *Ann Rheum Dis* **67**:1689–96.

PSORIATIC ARTHRITIS

Gladman D (2005). Traditional and newer therapeutic options for psoriatic arthritis: an evidence-based review. *Drugs* **65**:1223.

Ritchlin CT (2005). Pathogenesis of psoriatic arthritis. *Curr Opin Rheumatol* **17**:406.

INFLAMMATORY BOWEL DISEASE-ASSOCIATED ARTHRITIS

Ho P, Bruce I, Silman A, *et al*. (2005). Evidence for common genetic control in pathways of inflammation for Crohn's disease and psoriatic arthritis. *Arthritis Rheum* **52**:3596.

Wollheim F (2001). Enteropathic arthritis: how do the joints talk with the gut? *Curr Opin Rheumatol* **13**:305.

UVEITIS

Linder R, Hoffman A, Brunner R (2004). Prevalence of the spondyloarthritides in patients with uveitis. *J Rheumatol* **31**:2226–9.

Rosenbaum JT (2010). Future of biological therapy for uveitis. *Curr Opin Ophthalmol* 21:473–7.

Smith JA, Mackensen F, Sen HN, *et al*. (2009). Epidemiology and course of disease in childhood uveitis. *Opthalmology* **116**:1544–51.

BEHÇET'S DISEASE

Hatemi G, Silman A, Bang D, *et al*. (2009). Management of Behçet disease: a systematic literature review for the European League Against Rheumatism evidence-based recommendations for the management of Behçet disease. *Ann Rheum Dis* **68**:1528–34.

Yazici Y, Yurdakul S, Yazici H (2010). Behçet's syndrome. *Curr Rheumatol Rep* **12**:429–35.

Chapter 4
Juvenile Idiopathic Arthritis

JUVENILE IDIOPATHIC ARTHRITIS

Hashkes PJ, Laxer RM (2005). Medical treatment of juvenile idiopathic arthritis. *JAMA* **294**:1671–84.

Packham JC, Hall MA (2002). Long-term follow-up of 246 adults with juvenile idiopathic arthritis: functional outcome. *Rheumatology (Oxford)* **41**:1428–35.

Petty RE, Southwood TR, Manners P, *et al*. (2004). International league of associations for rheumatology classification of juvenile idiopathic arthritis: Second revision, Edmonton, 2001. *J Rheumatol* **31**:390–2.

HEREDITARY PERIODIC FEVERS

Henderson C, Goldbach-Mansky R (2010). Monogenic autoinflammatory diseases: new insights into clinical aspects and pathogenesis. *Curr Opin Rheumatol* **22**:567–78.

Kastner DL, Aksentijevich I, Goldbach-Mansky R (2010). Autoinflammatory disease reloaded: a clinical perspective. *Cell* **140**:784–90.

Chapter 5
Connective Tissue Diseases

RAYNAUD'S PHENOMEN

Boin F, Wigley FM (2005). Understanding, assessing and treating Raynaud's phenomenon. *Rheum Dis Clin North Am* **31**:465–81.

SJÖGREN'S SYNDROME

Fox RI, Saito I (1994). Criteria for diagnosis of Sjögren's syndrome. *Rheum Dis Clin North Am* **20**:391–407.

Mariette X, Gottenberg JE (2010). Pathogenesis of Sjögren's syndrome and therapeutic consequences. *Curr Opin Rheumatol* **22**:471–7.

Ramos-Casals M, Tzioufas AG, Stone JH, Siso A, Bosch X (2010). Treatment of primary Sjögren's syndrome: a systematic review. *JAMA* **304**:452–60.

SYSTEMIC LUPUS ERYTHEMATOSUS

Bertsias GK, Salmon JE, Boumpas DT (2010). Therapeutic opportunities in systemic lupus erythematosus: state of the art and prospects for the new decade. *Ann Rheum Dis* **69**:1603–11.

Boumpas DT, Austin HA, Vaughan EM, *et al*. (1992). Severe lupus nephritis: controlled trial of pulse methylprednisolone versus two different regimens of pulse cyclophosphamide. *Lancet* **340**:741–4.

Calvo-Alen J, Bastian HM, Straaton KV, Burgard SL, Mikhail IS, Alarcon GS (1995). Identification of patient subsets among those preemptively diagnosed with referred and/or followed up for systemic lupus erythematosus at a large tertiary care center. *Arthritis Rheum* **38**:1475–84.

Laman SD, Provost TT (1994). Cutaneous manifestations of lupus erythematosus. *Rheum Dis Clin North Am* **20**:195–212.

Manzi S, Seilahn EN, Rairie J, *et al*. (1997). Age-specific incidence rates of myocardial infarction and angina in women with system lupus erythematosus. *Am J Epidemiol* **145**:408–15.

Tan EM, Cohen AS, Fries JF, *et al*. (1982). The 1982 revised criteria for the classification of systemic lupus erythematosus. *Arthritis Rheum* **25**:1271–7.

West SG, Emlen W, Wener MH, Kotzin BL (1995). Neuropsychiatric lupus erythematosus: a 10-year prospective study on the value of diagnostic tests. *Am J Med* **99**:153–63.

DRUG-INDUCED LUPUS

Chang C, Gershwin ME (2010). Drugs and autoimmunity – a contemporary review and mechanistic approach. *J Autoimmun* **34**:J266–75.

ANTIPHOSPHOLIPID ANTIBODY SYNDROME

Cervera R, Piette JC, Font J, *et al*. (2002). Antiphospholipid syndrome: clinical and immunologic manifestations and patterns of disease expression in a cohort of 1,000 patients. *Arthritis Rheum* **46**:1019–27.

Crowther MA, Wisloff F (2005). Evidence based treatment of the antiphospholipid syndrome II. Optimal anticoagulant therapy for thrombosis. *Thromb Res* **115**(1–2):3–8.

POLYMYOSITIS AND DERMATOMYOSITIS

Bohan A, Peter JB (1975). Polymyositis and dermatomyositis (parts I and 2). *NEJM* **292**:344–7, 403–7.

Dalakas MC (1991). Polymyositis, dermatomyositis and inclusion-body myositis. *NEJM* **325**:1487–98.

Lotz BP, Engel AG, Nishino H, *et al*. (1989). Inclusion body myositis. Observations in 40 patients. *Brain* **112**:727–47.

McAdam LP, O'Hanlan MA, Bluestone R, Pearson CM (1976). Relapsing polychondritis: prospective study of 23 patients and review of the literature. *Medicine* (Baltimore) **55**:193–215.

Michet CJ, McKenna CH, Luthra HS, O'Fallon WM (1986). Relapsing polychondritis. Survival and predictive role of early manifestations. *Ann Intern Med* 104:74–8.

SYSTEMIC SCLEROSIS (SCLERODERMA)

Cheema GS, Quismorio Jr FP (2001). Interstitial lung disease in systemic sclerosis. *Curr Opin Pulm Med* 7:283–90.

DeMarco PJ, Weisman MH, Seibold JR, *et al*. (2002). Predictors and outcomes of scleroderma renal crisis: the high-dose versus low-dose D-penicillamine in early diffuse systemic sclerosis trial. *Arthritis Rheum* **46**(11):2983–9.

Kowal-Bielecka O, Landewe R, Avouac J, *et al*. (2009). EULAR recommendations for the treatment of systemic sclerosis: a report from the EULAR Scleroderma Trials and Research group (EUSTAR). Ann Rheum Dis **68**:620–8.

LeRoy EC, Black C, Fleischmajer R, *et al*. (1988). Scleroderma (systemic sclerosis): classification, subsets and pathogenesis. *J Rheumatol* **15**(2):202–5.

MacGregor AJ, Canavan R, Knight C, *et al*. (2001). Pulmonary hypertension in systemic sclerosis: risk factors for progression and consequences for survival. *Rheumatol* **40**(4):453–9.

Rose S, Young MA, Reynolds JC (1998). Gastrointestinal manifestations of scleroderma. *Gastroenterol Clin North Am* **27**:563–94.

MIXED CONNECTIVE TISSUE DISEASE AND UNDIFFERENTIATED CONNECTIVE TISSUE DISEASE

Burdt MA, Hoffman RW, Deutscher SL, Wang GS, Johnson JC, Sharp GC (1999). Longterm outcome in mixed connective tissue disease. *Arthritis Rheum* **42**:899–909.

Sharp GC, Irvin WS, Gould RG, Holman HR, Tan EM (1972). Mixed connective tissue disease. An apparently distinct rheumatic disease syndrome associated with a specific antibody to an extractable nuclear antigen (ENA). *Am J Med* **52**:148–59.

RELAPSING POLYCHONDRITIS

Lahmer T, Treiber M, von Werder A, *et al*. (2010). Relapsing polychondritis: an autoimmune disease with many faces. *Autoimmune Rev* 9:540–6

Chapter 6
Vasculitis

INTRODUCTION

Basu N, Watts R, Bajema I, *et al*. (2010). EULAR points to consider in the development of classification and diagnostic criteria in systemic vasculitis. *Ann Rheum Dis* 69:1744–50.

Langford CA (2010). Vasculitis. *J Allergy Clin Immunol* 125(2 suppl 2):S216–25.

GIANT CELL ARTERITIS AND POLYMYALGIA RHEUMATICA

Bongartz T, Matteson EL (2006). Large-vessel involvement in giant cell arteritis. *Curr Opin Rheumatol* 18(1):10–17.

Salvarani C, Cantini F, Boiardi L, Hunder GG (2002). Polymyalgia rheumatica and giant-cell arteritis. *NEJM* 347(4):261–71.

Weyand CM, Goronzy JJ (2003). Giant-cell arteritis and polymyalgia rheumatica. *Ann Intern Med* 139(6):505–15.

TAKAYASU'S ARTERITIS

Seo P, Stone JH (2004). Large-vessel vasculitis. *Arthritis Rheum* 51(1):128–39.

ANCA-ASSOCIATED VASCULITIS – WEGENER'S GRANULOMATOSIS, MICROSCOPIC POLYANGIITIS, AND CHURG–STRAUSS SYNDROME

Agard C, Mouthon L, Mahr A, Guillevin L (2003). Microscopic polyangiitis and polyarteritis nodosa: how and when do they start? *Arthritis Rheum* 49:709–15.

Cohen P, Pagnoux C, Mahr A, *et al*. (2007). Churg–Strauss syndrome with poor-prognosis factors: a prospective multicenter trial comparing glucocorticoids and six or twelve cyclophosphamide pulses in forty-eight patients. *Arthritis Rheum* 57:686–93.

Guillevin L, Cohen P, Mahr A, *et al*. (2003). Treatment of polyarteritis nodosa and microscopic polyangiitis with poor-prognosis factors: a prospective trial comparing glucocorticoids and six or twelve cyclophosphamide pulses in sixty-five patients. *Arthritis Rheum* 49:93–100.

Keogh KA, Specks U (2006). Churg–Strauss syndrome: update on clinical, laboratory and therapeutic aspects. *Sarcoidosis Vasc Diffuse Lung Dis* 23:3–12.

Langford CA, Talar-Willams C, Barron KS, Sneller MC (2003). Use of acyclophosphamide–induction, methotrexate-maintenance regimen for the treatment of Wegener's granulomatosis: extended follow-up and rate of relapse. *Am J Med* 114:463–9.

Stone JH, Merkel PA, Spiera R, *et al*. (2010). Rituximab versus cyclophosphamide for ANCA-associated vasculitis. *NEJM* 363:221–32.

POLYARTERITIS NODOSA

Guillevin L, Mahr A, Callard P, *et al*. (2005). Hepatitis B virus-associated polyarteritis nodosa: clinical characteristics, outcome, and impact of treatment in 115 patients. *Medicine (Baltimore)* 84:313–22.

Selga D, Mohammad A, Sturfelt G, Segelmark M (2006). Polyarteritis nodosa when applying the Chapel Hill nomenclature: a descriptive study on ten patients. *Rheumatology (Oxford)* 45:1276–81.

Stone JH (2002). Polyarteritis nodosa. *JAMA* 288:1632–9.

IMMUNE COMPLEX-MEDIATED SMALL-VESSEL VASCULITIS

Ballinger S (2003). Henoch-Schönlein purpura. *Curr Opin Rheumatol* 15(5):591–4.

Carslson JA, Cavaliere LF, Grant-Kels JM (2006). Cutaneous vasculitis: diagnosis and management. *Clin Dermatol* 24:414–29.

Ferri C, Mascia MT (2006). Cryoglobulinemic vasculitis. *Curr Opin Rheumatol* 18(1):54–63.

KAWASAKI'S DISEASE

Burns JC, Glode MP (2004). Kawasaki syndrome. *Lancet* 364:533–44.

Oates-Whitehead RM, Baumer JH, Haines L, *et al*. (2003). Intravenous immunoglobulin for the treatment of Kawasaki disease in children. *Cochrane Database Syst Rev* 2(4):CD004000.

THROMBOANGIITIS OBLITERANS (BUERGER'S DISEASE)

Olin JW, Shih A (2006). Thromboangiitis obliterans (Buerger's disease). *Curr Opin Rheumatol* 18(1):18–24.

PRIMARY ANGIITIS OF THE CENTRAL NERVOUS SYSTEM

Calabrese LH, Mallek JA (1988). Primary angiitis of the central nervous system. Report of 8 new cases, review of the literature, and proposal for diagnostic criteria. *Medicine* (Baltimore) 67:20–39.

Calabrese LH, Molloy ES, Singhal AB (2007). Primary central nervous system vasculitis: progress and questions. *Ann Neurol* **62**:430–2.

Salvarani C, Brown RD, Calamia KT, *et al*. (2007). Primary central nervous system vasculitis: analysis of 101 patients. *Ann Neurol* **62**:442–51.

Chapter 7
Other Rheumatic Conditions

OSTEOPOROSIS

Grossman JM, Gordon R, Ranganath VK, *et al*. (2010). American College of Rheumatology 2010 recommendations for the prevention and treatment of glucocorticoid-induced osteoporosis. *Arthritis Care Res (Hoboken)* **62**:1515–26.

Schett G, Saag KG, Bijlsma JW (2010). From bone biology to clinical outcome: state of the art and future perspectives. *Ann Rheum Dis* **69**:1415–9.

FIBROMYALGIA AND OTHER SOFT TISSUE SYNDROMES

Busch A, Schachter CL, Peloso PM, Bombardier C (2002). Exercise for treating fibromyalgia syndrome. *Cochrane Database Syst Rev* CD003786.

Crofford LJ (2008). Pain management in fibromyalgia. *Curr Opin Rheumatol* **20**:246–50.

Wallace DJ (1997). The fibromyalgia syndrome. *Ann Med* **29**:9–21.

Wolfe F, Smythe HA, Yunnus MB, *et al*. (1990). The American College of Rheumatology 1990 criteria for the classification of fibromyalgia: Report of the Multicenter Criteria Committee. *Arthritis Rheum* **33**:160–72.

SARCOIDOSIS

Chatham W (2010). Rheumatic manifestations of systemic disease: sarcoidosis. *Curr Opin Rheumatol* **22**:85–90.

Newman LS, Rose CS, Maier LA (1997). Sarcoidosis. *NEJM* **336**:1224–34.

Sweiss NJ, Patterson K, Sawaqed R, *et al*. (2010). Rheumatologic manifestations of sarcoidosis. *Semin Respir Crit Care Med* **31**:463–73.

AMYLOIDOSIS

Falk RH, Comenzo RL, Skinner M (1997). The systemic amyloidoses. *NEJM* **337**:898–909.

Kyle RA, Gertz MA (1995). Primary systemic amyloidosis: clinical and laboratory features in 474 cases. *Semin Hematol* **32**:45–59.

MISCELLANEOUS RHEUMATIC CONDITIONS

Bland JH, Frymoyer JW, Newberg AH, *et al*. (1979). Rheumatic syndromes in endocrine disease. *Semin Arthritis Rheum* **9**:23–65.

Naschitz JE, Rosner I, Rozenbaum M, *et al*. (1995). Cancer associated rheumatic disorders: clues to occult neoplasia. *Semin Arthritis Rheum* **24**:231–4.

Naschitz JE, Yeshurun D, Rosner I (1995). Rheumatic manifestations of occult cancer. *Cancer* **75**:2954–8.

Sequeira W (1994). The neuropathic joint. *Clin Exper Rheumatol* **12**:325–37.

Index

Note: Page numbers in *italic* refer to tables or boxes